THE MEDITERRANEAN DIET

ROCKRIDGE
UNIVERSITY PRESS

ISBN: Print 978-1-62315-100-3 | eBook 978-1-62315-005-1

CONTENTS

INTRODUCTION

These days, there seems to be a new diet making headlines every time you pick up a magazine or turn on the television. Weight loss is big business. Obesity is at an all-time high, and the negative health effects of being overweight are clear. Diets that promise an easier, faster way to lose weight are more popular than ever, and everyone is scrambling to create the newest best seller. Ironically, the most respected and successful diets have been around for centuries. If you're looking for a time-tested, healthful eating regimen filled with delicious foods, you've found it in the Mediterranean diet.

The Mediterranean diet is a way of eating that is common among the coastal areas of Greece, Italy, and Spain. It hasn't changed much over the years, but it's recently gotten a great deal of attention from the medical community, nutrition professionals, media, and dieters. It isn't new science and it isn't rocket science. It isn't about counting calories, measuring grams, or combining foods in just the "right" way at just the "right" time. Furthermore, the Mediterranean diet isn't just about *what* the Mediterranean people eat, but about *how* they eat.

The Mediterranean diet focuses on fruits and vegetables, whole grains, nuts, legumes, and fish, with the occasional red meat, poultry, and dairy—almost a complete reverse from the standard American diet. Equally as important on the Mediterranean diet is eating locally and seasonally, as well as consciously. While Americans tend to eat on the run, in front of TV or computers, and distracted, Mediterraneans take time to savor each meal, usually with friends and family. By paying attention to everything they eat, Mediterraneans savor flavors and are much less likely than Americans to grab a convenient but tasteless processed food, which means they are much less likely to eat junk food, saturated fats, and empty calories.

In short, the Mediterranean diet is for people to actually love to eat. Sound good? Read on!

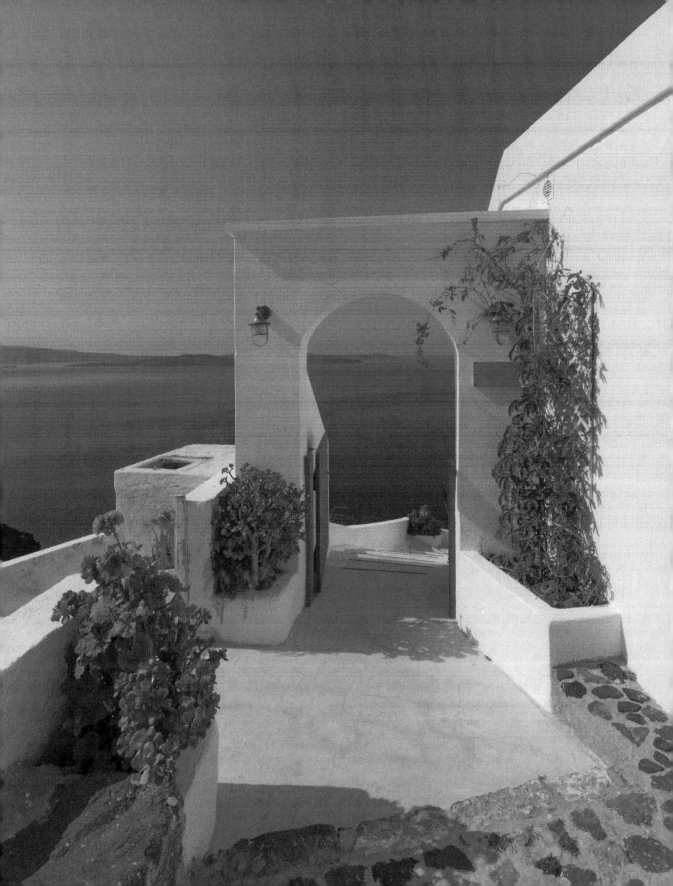

SECTION ONE:

The Basics of the Mediterranean Diet

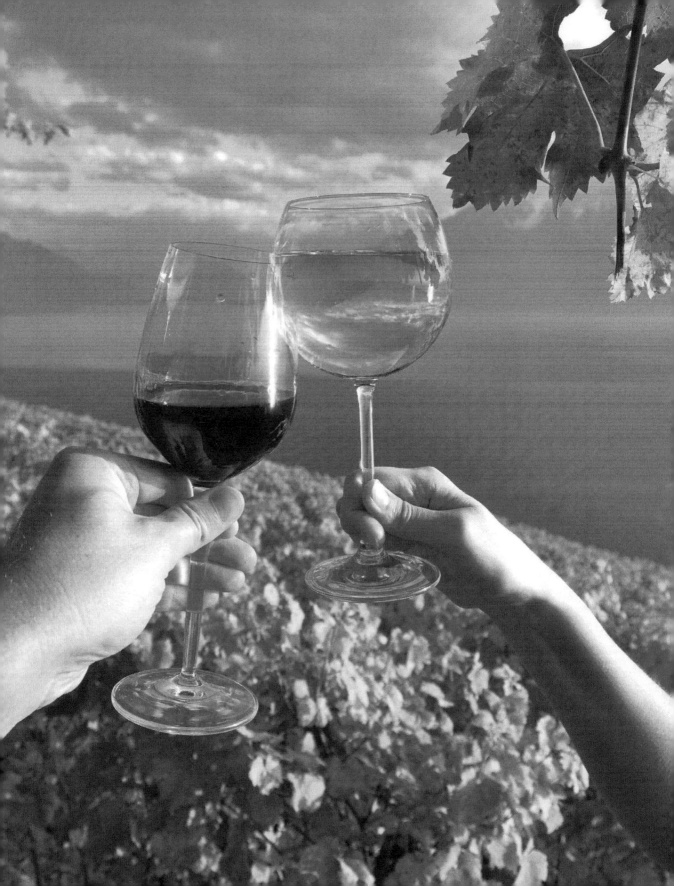

$$\left(\begin{array}{c} 1 \end{array}\right)$$

WHAT THE MEDITERRANEAN DIET WILL DO FOR YOU

According to the respected Mayo Clinic, the Mediterranean diet reduces overall heart-related deaths, incidence of cancer and cancer-related deaths, and incidences of Parkinson's and Alzheimer's diseases. Do you need more reasons? Good, because there are plenty more; by following the Mediterranean diet, you'll:

- Improve heart and artery health
- Improve moods and mental function
- Improve the look and feel of your skin
- Increase energy
- Lower high blood pressure
- Lower LDL (bad) cholesterol and raise HDL (good) cholesterol
- Reduce body fat and lose excess weight
- Reduce your chances of developing type 2 diabetes

Not only does the Mediterranean diet do all of this, it does so without costing you a fortune, sucking up your time, or complicating your (already complicated) life.

How can the Mediterranean diet be attributed with so many health benefits? One of the biggest reasons is the fact that the Mediterranean diet cuts out unhealthful, saturated fats and uses a lot of healthful, polyunsaturated fats.

The Mediterraneans eat very little meat and almost no fast food or prepackaged food—most saturated fats occur in animal products and processed foods—so they get very little saturated fat in their daily diet. However, the diet is high in polyunsaturated fats. In fact,

Mediterraneans' total daily fat intake is higher than most popular diets recommend and yet they are healthier and slimmer. This is because it isn't so much *how much fat* you eat as it is *what kind of fat* you eat.

The polyunsaturated fats common in the Mediterranean diet actually lower bad cholesterol, improve heart and artery health, create smoother, more youthful skin, increase energy, and even improve mood and mental function.

While these healthful fats can help you have more energy, the increased intake of vitamins, minerals, and phytonutrients from all that fresh produce will give you more energy than you can believe. And because you'll lose excess pounds, especially around the abdomen, you'll also greatly reduce your chances of developing type 2 diabetes.

Natural Weight Loss

Of course, you not only want to be healthy, you also want to lose weight and maintain a healthful weight easily. The Mediterranean diet will enable you to do that, and you won't have to count calories, worry about food combinations, or carry a calculator and scale to work with you.

Because you won't be eating fast food, deep-fried foods, or heavily processed foods, you'll be cutting out an enormous number of calories without even trying.

Additionally, you'll be adding a huge amount of vitamins, fiber, antioxidants, and omega-3s that will help you to feel full and satisfied and even help you burn stored fat, especially around the abdomen.

By eating the Mediterranean diet, you'll be enjoying healthful foods that promote heart and artery health, improve mental function, stabilize mood, and improve skin tone and texture; losing weight will be a happy by-product. Of course, if your priority is losing weight, you can step it up by following the guidelines in the next chapter.

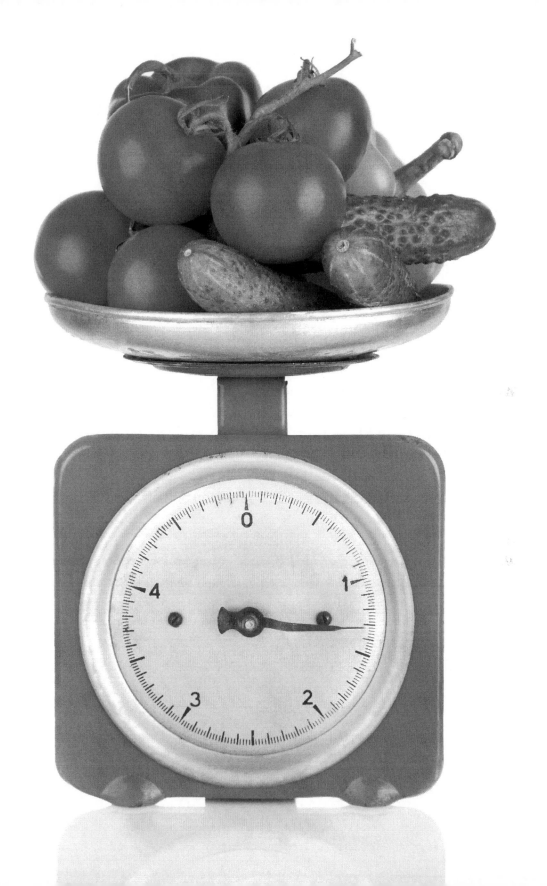

(2)

HOW TO LOSE WEIGHT ON THE MEDITERRANEAN DIET

Although the Mediterranean diet was first recognized for its extremely healthful way of eating, it didn't take long for people to notice that it was also a safe, healthful, and effective way to lose weight. If weight loss is a big part of your motivation in undertaking the Mediterranean diet, you won't be disappointed.

The Mediterranean diet, by its nature, lends itself quite easily to almost mindless weight loss. If that sounds too good to be true, read on. The Mediterranean Diet Pyramid is largely made up of foods that are water-rich and high in fiber. (For more on the Mediterranean Diet Pyramid, see the next chapter.) This means that they fill you up quickly without adding a lot of calories. The diet also includes lots of healthful, lean protein and unsaturated fats, as well as many nutrients and micronutrients that actually aid in the process of using up or metabolizing stored fat, especially in the abdominal area.

Because of this, you will likely find yourself losing weight without counting calories or having to think too much about it. Most people who go on the Mediterranean diet can expect to lose between two and five pounds per week, as long as they follow some simple guidelines. More important, you'll be building healthful habits that will benefit your heart health, blood pressure, blood sugar, and insulin regulation.

The Mediterranean way of life is low-stress, low-key, and enjoyable. Your diet should be, too, and that's one of the things that make the Mediterranean diet so wonderful.

Planning Your Diet

Once you've read through this book and you know what foods you should be eating and what foods you shouldn't, make a list of the foods you want to include in your weekly diet. In other words, don't think you have to eat every allowable food on the Mediterranean diet. If you don't like eggplant, there's no intelligent reason for you to eat it. When you look at the fish and seafood recommended on the diet, choose the ones that appeal to you and are affordable and readily available.

The foods that are a part of the Mediterranean diet are so varied and plentiful that you'll have lots of choices when it's time to plan your diet and your daily meals. You don't need to limit yourself to "Mediterranean" foods or Italian or Greek dishes, either. You can eat Japanese meals, French meals, and plain old American dishes on the Mediterranean diet. It's all about choosing the right ingredients, preparing them the right way, and following a few lifestyle guidelines.

Eat Small Meals All Day Long

It is widely known that you will lose weight faster, feel full longer, have more energy, and keep your blood sugar steady if you eat several small meals a day, rather than two or three large ones. When you skip meals, your blood sugar and energy levels plummet, your body screams for fuel, and you end up eating a lot more than you should and usually a lot of something you shouldn't be eating at all.

On the Mediterranean diet, especially if your goal is to lose weight, you want to eat at least every two hours. This doesn't mean a full three-course dinner or even a full plate every two hours. What you need is a healthful meal, mini-meal, or snack every two to three hours. This could be a stick of mozzarella cheese and a pear, a smoothie, or your evening meal.

The best way to ensure that you eat well and often enough is to make good choices accessible. Spend a few minutes making a huge fruit salad of melons, strawberries, kiwis, grapes, and apples, and you'll have a cup or container of delicious fruit anytime you need it during the week.

Fill a container with your favorite vegetables sliced up, make small bags of nuts and dried fruits to take to work, and keep your blender out on the counter for whipping up quick shakes and smoothies.

The easier it is to grab a quick mini-meal or snack, the more likely you are to keep your hunger at bay, no matter where you are or what time it is.

Think More about Portions, Less about Calories

The Mediterranean way of eating includes snacks made up of two or three simple, fresh foods and meals that take place over several small courses. In America, people think of a meal as a heaping plate filled with everything that's on the table. In the Mediterranean, people enjoy one part of the meal at a time.

They may start with a small plate of green salad or roasted peppers, savor a small bowl of delicious soup, move on to a delectable filet of fish on a bed of rice, then enjoy some cheese and fruit for dessert. This way of eating is all about enjoying each portion of the meal for what it is, rather than lumping everything together and rushing through it.

The terrific bonus to this way of eating is that you end up eating a lot less and enjoying it more. It takes approximately twenty minutes for your stomach to signal that it's full. In that time, most Americans will have already eaten way more than they should. By the time their stomachs notice they're eating, they've already overeaten.

If you change your pattern to eating smaller portions in a course-by-course meal, you'll already be starting to feel satisfied before you've gotten to the main part of your meal. Therefore, you'll eat far less.

At first, try focusing on your portions and the time you take to eat, rather than looking at how many calories you're taking in. After a week or so, if your weight loss isn't as fast as you'd like it to be, go ahead and follow these guidelines for speeding up your weight loss by taking in fewer calories and burning more.

However, keep in mind that just the stress of counting calories can stimulate the release of the stress hormone cortisol. Cortisol responds to stress by directing the storage of fat in the abdominal area. Counting calories can actually make you gain weight!

Tips for Success

Prepare Your Pantry

Make a copy of the foods list and the food pyramid that appears later in this book and stick it on your fridge. It'll help you plan your shopping and your meals and snacks, without having to look everything up each time.

Before you get started on your diet, go through your pantry, fridge, and cupboards and get rid of any lurking land mines. If you live alone or with a spouse that will also be on the diet, that makes it easier; just give away or throw away anything that's not allowable, such as margarine, donuts, frozen French fries, etc. If you have a family that will not be following the diet, designate a certain cupboard and a particular refrigerator shelf for forbidden foods, then stay away from it.

Try Something New Once a Week

If you've never been much of a vegetable eater, you may be tempted to stick to the broccoli, carrots, and green beans you usually eat. If fish has never featured prominently in your diet, you may get stuck looking for new ways to eat tuna. Don't limit yourself to the things you've always eaten. The Mediterranean people have a huge taste for adventure and discovery that extends to their diets. You should, too.

At least once a week, try a food you've never eaten. You might hate it, but more times than not, you'll find yourself enjoying something new and exotic (at least, exotic to you).

This can really liven up your diet, make shopping more fun, and help prevent boredom with the diet. The foods allowed on the Mediterranean diet are so vast and varied, there's simply no excuse for being bored.

So, try a slice of papaya, some falafel, or roasted eggplant dip. You never know, you just might love it, and you have nothing to lose if you don't.

Drink Plenty of Water

This is advice that many dieters are tired of hearing, but getting enough water is not only essential to good health, it's one of the key factors in losing weight, for a number of reasons:

- Your body needs plenty of water to get rid of stored fat and toxins.
- Many hunger pangs are actually thirst. Drink a glass of water if you find yourself searching for something to eat but don't know what—it usually means you're not hungry at all, just thirsty. If you're still hungry ten minutes later, go ahead and eat.
- You'll likely be eating a great deal more fiber than you're used to. Getting plenty of water ensures that that fiber moves through your system efficiently. The bonus: it's going to take a lot of fat and other foes with it.

Aim for a minimum of sixty-four ounces of water per day, more if you spend a great deal of time out in the heat or are working out regularly. If you're one of the many people who have a hard time drinking enough water, try freezing bottled water and take the frozen bottles with you to work, the gym, or in the car. Many people find ice-cold water much more palatable and you won't be so tempted to grab a soda from the office vending machine.

If plain water makes you curl up your lip, try adding slices of citrus fruit, a squeeze of lemon juice, or some berries to your water. It may be enough to make it more refreshing and appetizing for you, without adding the sugar and calories of bottled, flavored waters.

Follow Your Cravings

This sounds like bad advice, but it isn't. Your body was designed to ask for what it needs. The problem arises when people muddy the waters with their habits and addictions, such as eating in front of the TV because they always have, or reaching for cookies when they want something sweet.

If you're craving a salty snack, you likely need a bit more sodium or other minerals in your diet. If you're craving citrus, your body may be nagging for the vitamin C so essential to every one of your body's cells. A craving for steak may indicate you're not getting enough protein.

Fill your pantry, fridge, and desk drawer with healthful choices in all of the food groups, then follow your cravings. As you learn to listen to what your body is saying, you'll eventually start reaching for fruit instead of cookies when you need a quick pick-me-up.

Snack from the Bottom Up

Staring into the fridge and you don't know what you want? Already had a glass of water? Grab something from the bottom of the Mediterranean Food Pyramid first, which is fresh fruits and vegetables. Aim for something that's high in water and fiber content, like a slice of watermelon or an orange. It'll fill you up faster and longer. If you're still hungry, reach for the next food group, grains. If that doesn't satisfy you, move on up to the proteins. Eventually, you'll be satisfied, but by starting at the bottom, you'll take in fewer calories while you're trying to hit the spot.

Calories and Other Math

If you want to speed up your weight loss efforts, or if dieting without counting calories sounds too vague for you, you can follow a more traditional weight loss plan.

For every pound per week you want to lose, you'll have to get rid of 3,500 calories, or 500 calories a day. The healthiest and least painful way to do this is to burn half and just not eat the other half. In other words, cut your daily diet by 250 calories, burn another 250 per day, and you'll typically lose one pound per week. Cut 500 calories per day and burn another 500, and you'll typically lose two pounds per week.

This is not taking into consideration the weight you'll lose from water build-up, toxins, and stored fat that is now being metabolized. It's possible to burn one to two pounds more per week than you're planning.

In order to cut your calories, you need to know how many you're taking in or should be taking in to maintain your weight. For an exact number, you can use one of many calorie calculators on the Internet. For a pretty good estimate, multiply your weight by twelve to calculate your daily calorie allotment. For example, if you weigh 150 pounds, you require somewhere around 1,800 calories per day to maintain that weight. In this example, to lose one pound a week by dieting alone, set your daily intake to 1,300. If you want to be able to enjoy more calories, cut your calories to 1,550 per day and do 250 calories worth of exercise (a thirty-minute brisk walk will do it) per day. You'll get to eat more, but you'll still lose one pound per week.

Do not cut your calories too low. Not only is it unhealthful, but it won't work. Anything below 1,200 calories per day for women or 1,800 calories for men will result in an almost immediate slowing of the metabolism. You'll burn fewer calories throughout the day and actually add stored fat from the foods you eat. You'll also be miserable, grumpy, fatigued, and starving. Eating many small meals a day that include the foods allowed on the Mediterranean diet will rev up your metabolism. This allows you to lose more weight faster than starving yourself. There's no reason for you to put yourself on a strict deprivation plan.

What You Can Expect to Lose

As previously stated, you can target losing two or more pounds per week on the Mediterranean diet without counting calories or putting a great deal of thought into it. If you step that up with some moderate daily exercise, you'll lose weight faster, increase your heart and bone health, and reshape your body at the same time.

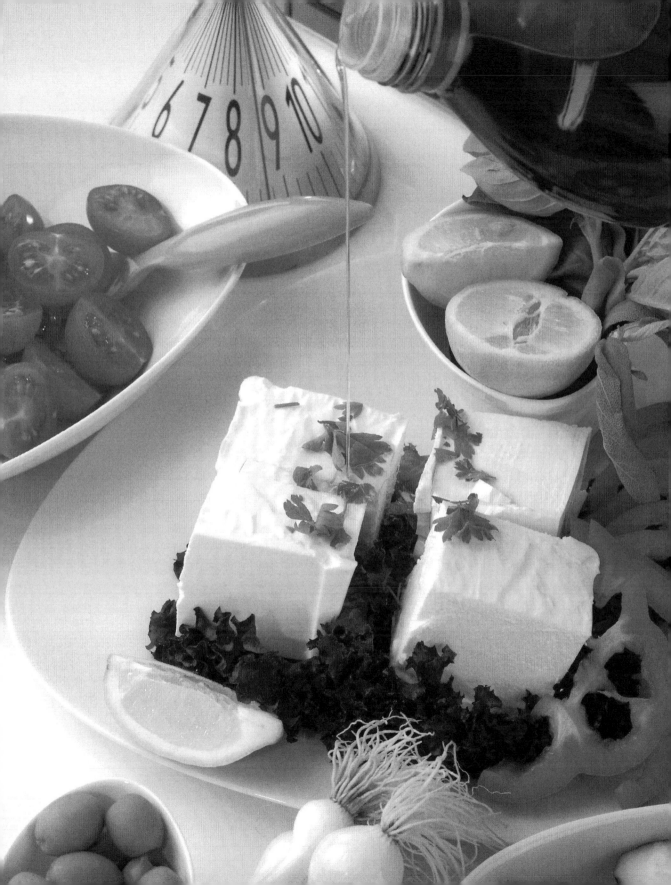

(3)

THE MEDITERRANEAN DIET FOOD GUIDE

Many people embarking on the Mediterranean diet assume that they'll have to eat mainly Greek, Middle Eastern, or Italian foods, but this isn't so.

While you can certainly check out some great dishes from Mediterranean cuisines and probably find some new favorite meals, you don't need to limit yourself to these types of foods. The Mediterranean diet is all about making healthful choices from a huge variety of delicious foods. You can follow the Mediterranean diet while eating Spanish food, Japanese food, or American food.

This probably comes as a relief to those of you who are too busy or on too tight a budget to troll the specialty grocers looking for grape leaves, quinoa, pine nuts, or ground spring lamb.

When reading through the Mediterranean diet food guidelines, keep these principles in mind:

- Don't eat anything just because it's on the list. These are the foods you can and should eat, not the foods you have to eat.
- On the other hand, be open to trying at least one new food a week. It'll keep things interesting and widen your choices as you strive to eat seasonally and locally.
- The key word is variety. You need a lot of it to have a balanced and interesting diet.
- Give yourself the most choices from the groups toward the bottom of the pyramid. If you're eating beef only once a month, you probably won't get bored with your favorite steak. However, when you're eating several fruits and vegetables a day, it's a good idea to have a wide choice.

The Mediterranean Food Pyramid

The food pyramid for the Mediterranean diet is very different from the daily diet that most Americans follow. The American diet is generally loaded with meats, processed flour and grains, sugar, and trans fats. The Mediterranean diet is almost an inverted version of that typical food pyramid.

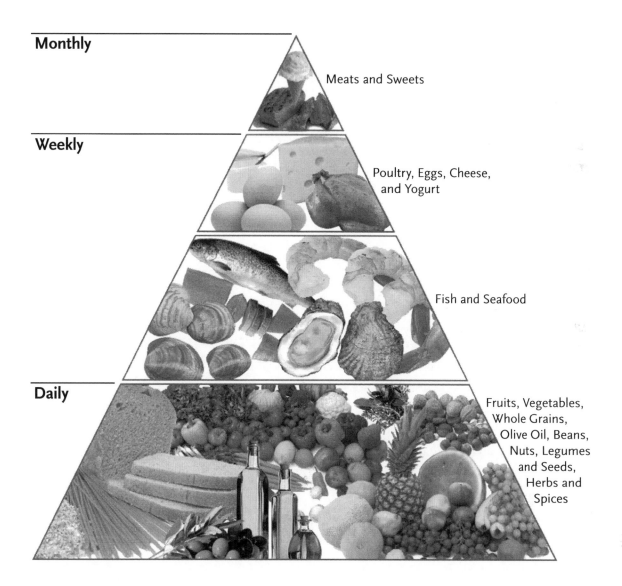

Monthly — Meats and Sweets

Weekly — Poultry, Eggs, Cheese, and Yogurt

Fish and Seafood

Daily — Fruits, Vegetables, Whole Grains, Olive Oil, Beans, Nuts, Legumes and Seeds, Herbs and Spices

As you can see, the foundation of the Mediterranean pyramid is divided between whole grains, legumes and nuts, and fruits and vegetables. In this example, the picture is even divided to show how often each food group is eaten.

In addition to grains, nuts, legumes, fruits, and vegetables, olive oil and dairy products such as cheese, yogurt, and milk make up the majority of the daily diet. This makes the Mediterranean daily diet one that is rich in healthful fats, fiber, protein, vitamins, and minerals.

In Mediterranean countries, fish, poultry, eggs, and sweets are typically eaten once or twice weekly. Meats such as pork, beef, and lamb are special meals that are eaten once only a month or so. It's an excellent idea for you to limit them to once or twice a month, as well. Animal products are the source of saturated fats, and saturated fats are what you need to avoid.

A glass of red wine is enjoyed after some meals but is rarely overindulged. If you don't care for wine or do not drink, pure grape juice from either red or Concord grapes is an excellent substitute that contains the many beneficial micronutrients of red wine.

Water is the beverage of preference, and a good deal of it is consumed on a daily basis.

This pattern of eating may have been started because of limited availability or finances, but it has remained the norm because it is a delicious, healthful way to eat.

Choosing the Best of the Best

Grains

The key to eating the best of the best grains is to choose whole-grain foods. They contain the fiber and natural goodness so integral to the Mediterranean diet.

Choose dense, heavy, chewy breads made from whole wheat, barley, and oats. Choose whole-grain pastas, too. Steel-cut, whole-grain oatmeal and multi-grain hot cereals are an excellent way to get your grains and stay satisfied all morning. If you like rice, opt for brown rice over white. Couscous, quinoa, and polenta are also good choices.

Fruits and Vegetables

Think color. A wide variety of dark red and orange vegetables and fruits provides many of the antioxidants and phytonutrients that are common to today's "super foods." These include red peppers, carrots, eggplant, sweet potatoes, tomatoes, and beets. Dark green leafy vegetables are also nutritional powerhouses. Be sure to eat plenty of spinach, kale, romaine lettuce, broccoli, bok choy, collards, and mustard and turnip greens.

All vegetables are allowed on the Mediterranean diet, but corn and white potatoes should be eaten in very limited quantities, as they contain far more starch than you need to consume on a regular basis. Some great choices are asparagus, zucchini, summer and winter squash, artichoke, green beans, and cauliflower, but with the Mediterranean diet, any veggie is a good veggie.

As with vegetables, you have free rein when choosing fruits. However, try to choose a wide variety of dark-colored fruits for their extraordinary nutritional punch. If you can, get plenty of blueberries, red raspberries, blackberries, red grapes, cranberries, and plums.

It's also a good idea to get plenty of fruits that contain a lot of water and fiber, such as watermelon, apples, oranges, and peaches. The extra water and fiber will help you feel satisfied longer and will also aid digestion.

Nuts and Legumes

The legumes you can choose from on the Mediterranean diet are limitless: eat split peas, black-eyed peas, kidney beans, black beans, great northern beans, or anything else you enjoy. Legumes provide a wealth of filling fiber, very little fat, and a lot of flavor. Try adding beans to your favorite soups and stews.

Be careful when choosing nuts and seeds for your diet. Some nuts are higher in unhealthful fats than others. These include peanuts, Brazil nuts, and cashews. Instead, stick with choices like almonds and walnuts. They're rich in omega-3s and taste great. When selecting nuts, it's best to opt for raw, unsalted nuts. If you don't care for raw nuts, go ahead and eat the toasted variety, but forgo the salt, honey-roasted or chocolate coatings!

Milk and Dairy Products

Goat and sheep's milk products are a lot more popular in the Mediterranean than they are here, but you certainly don't have to eat them if you don't care for the taste. The important thing is to choose low-fat varieties of milk and cheese and to not go overboard.

Yogurt is a very important part of the daily diet for most people in the Mediterranean, as are hard and soft cheeses. However, cheese isn't used heavily in meals. Cheese and fruit is a common dessert combination, and cheese is used to flavor and enhance food rather than overwhelm it.

If you're going to eat yogurt, go Greek. Greek yogurt has twice the protein of regular commercial yogurt. It's widely available in most supermarkets and has a rich, silky texture that you'll love. Bonus: it's usually about the same price as name-brand regular yogurt.

Fish and Seafood

Seafood is an integral part of the Mediterranean diet and accounts for much of its heart-healthful reputation. They're rich in omega-3s and other unsaturated fats, without all of the artery-clogging saturated fat of animal meats.

The best fish to choose is a cold-water variety, such as mackerel, cod, haddock, salmon, or sardines, because of their high content of omega-3s. However all fish is allowed on the diet.

In addition to fish, there are mussels, oysters, clams, crab, scallops, shrimp, and lobster from which to choose.

Fats and Oils

Most of the fats in the Mediterranean diet come directly from the foods and olive oils themselves. Butter is very rarely used and isn't missed. Canola oil may be used for some things that don't particularly suit the flavor of olive oil. Choose extra-virgin olive oil in a light version for salad dressings, and use on raw foods or in baking. Regular extra-virgin olive oil is fine for cooking. Don't feel that you have to go to a specialty store and buy an expensive bottle of oil. Buy the best supermarket variety that you can comfortably afford. Keep in mind, though, that you won't be using butter or margarine, so you'll be saving money there.

Sweets

For the most part, the people of the Mediterranean enjoy fruit and cheese after a meal as a sweet treat. You should try it; it's not only healthful but also delicious and light. For those times when you need a little something decadent, enjoy some dark chocolate (high in antioxidants), sorbet, sherbet, or Italian ice. Frozen yogurt is another nice option, as long as it's low-fat and not loaded with toppings that pack on sugar, fat, and calories.

Poultry and Meats

Poultry, beef, pork, and lamb are eaten only once or twice a month in most Mediterranean homes. You may need to slowly wean yourself from hamburgers, thick steaks, and pork chops, but this is a necessary step to reduce the unhealthful saturated fats that affect your heart, arteries, and body fat ratio. Lowering saturated fats is key to following the Mediterranean way of eating.

When you do have a meat dish, try these principles for getting the meat you want without hurting your diet:

- Choose organic meats.
- Choose the leanest cuts and trim any visible fat.
- Steer clear of all ground meats—even the "lean" ones are too high in fat and low in nutrients.
- Watch your portions. The leanest cultural groups in the world use meat as a flavoring, not as the star of a meal.

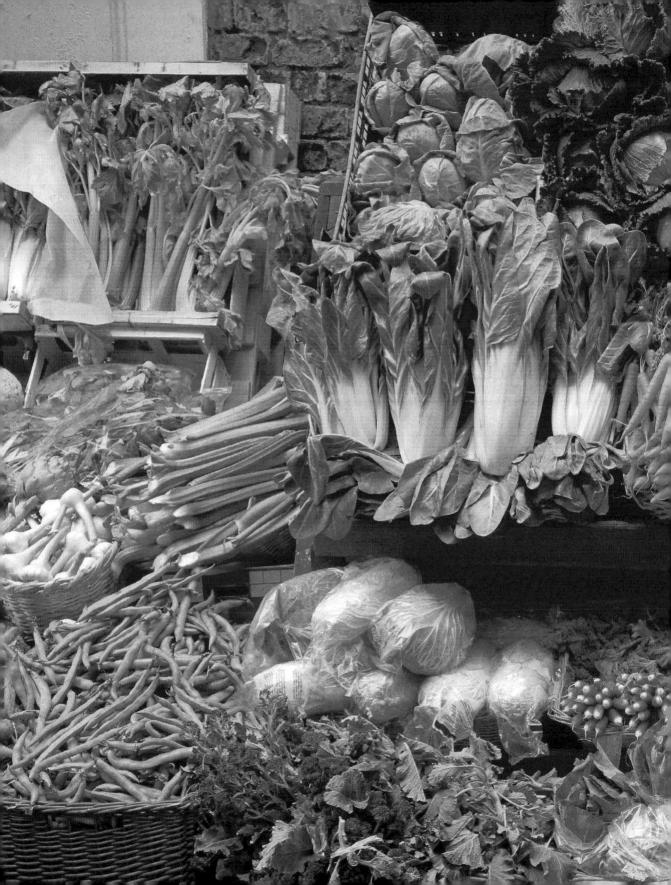

$$\left(\; 4 \; \right)$$

ADAPTING TO THE MEDITERRANEAN DIET AND LIFESTYLE

As stated before, the Mediterranean diet is as much about what foods you eat as it is about the lifestyle associated with the diet. Just as the choices you make at each meal can positively impact your health, so too can the choices you make throughout the day. Use the following guidelines to get the most out of the Mediterranean diet.

Eat Locally

The people of the Mediterranean region eat as many healthful, agricultural cultures have eaten for centuries: they eat what is available in their region at a given time.

What this means is that their food is as fresh as possible and usually produced without chemicals that are bad for your health.

To adopt this way of eating, shop as much as possible from local purveyors. Farmers' markets offer a huge selection of foods, from the freshest possible produce to organic honey and syrup and even meats and seafood. Does this mean you can never have a mango unless you go on vacation? Of course not. Nothing about the Mediterranean diet or the Mediterranean way of eating is rigid and joyless. Follow the principles as much as is realistic and enjoyable. Not everyone lives in the tropics.

To supplement what you get at the farmers' market, you can shop local artisan bakeries, health food stores, organic markets, and local butchers and seafood shops that have locally produced products.

If this sounds like a lot of running around to you, you can also specifically seek out locally grown or produced foods in your regular supermarket. At the very least, choose organic when you can.

Eat Seasonally

This goes hand in hand with eating locally. If you're getting most of your food from providers of locally grown items, you will be eating seasonal foods for the most part. Why is this important? What do the Mediterraneans know that Americans may not?

Eating foods when they're in season not only assures you food that is at its delicious peak, it also gets you in step with the seasons of food. People have grown so used to having watermelon and strawberries available all year long that they've lost the joy of something coming into its season. Watermelon is never more of a treat than it is in the heat of a July afternoon. Peas are supposed to be a sweet harbinger of spring, not a mealy pile dumped out of a can.

Eating seasonally, whenever possible and as much as possible, gets you in tune with the rhythm of food in the way that agricultural people and many Europeans have always been. This is a fun way to eat; it brings more joy to the table and to the mouth. It's also cheaper, since seasonal food is more abundant. Eat seasonally: your pocketbook and your waist will thank you.

Eat Consciously

As mentioned earlier, the people of the Mediterranean eat very consciously. They rarely eat while watching TV, driving, working, or reading. When they eat, they focus on the food and give themselves every reason to enjoy it.

Because of this, they eat less (they don't eat mindlessly, therefore they seldom overeat) and enjoy what they eat so much more.

Start by focusing solely on the meal or snack while you're eating. Don't eat while you're doing something else. If you need a quick bite at work, give yourself five or ten minutes to actually taste a handful of nuts, rather than popping them unnoticed into your mouth.

For meals and even small snacks, set yourself a nice table. Put a daisy in a vase, use a pretty plate, put on some soft music, or eat out on the patio. Even an apple can be more of an event when you eat it on a park bench instead of standing in front of a computer or munching on the interstate.

Eat Joyously

This is difficult for some Americans to grasp. The people of the Mediterranean love food. They love eating it and they love sharing it. Even simple meals have the feel of a celebration.

Start focusing on the ingredients in the dish before you. Close your eyes when you bite into that homegrown peach. smell it, taste it, and feel it. You'd be amazed at how much you don't notice about what you eat every day.

Whenever you can, eat with a loved one, a friend, or a group of people you really enjoy. Focus on the freshness and deliciousness of the food. Try new things together. Laugh as much as possible. There are a lot of reasons that Mediterraneans have so much less stress and stress-related illness. The fact that they really take joy in eating is one of them. They take their time, make the most of what they have, and enjoy the people around them.

Eating joyously is so different from the traditional experience of dieting. The thought of dieting usually conjures up deprivation, celery sticks, water, hunger, and resentment. The Mediterranean diet is a way to lose weight, get incredibly healthy, and have a great time, too.

Overworked, Overstressed, and Overscheduled

Even though the Mediterranean diet stresses sitting down and really enjoying your food, even when snacking, breakfast may be a difficult time for you to do that. However, using some shortcuts and compromises is far better than skipping the morning meal. There are some great smoothie recipes later in the book that you can use to have a healthful meal while getting ready for work or getting the kids out the door.

If you're running from the time you get up to the time you go to bed, invest in some of the pre-packaged snacks that work well with the Mediterranean diet, such as apples and yogurt, pre-cut veggies and fruit chunks, or small packs of nuts and dried fruits. If you have time, spend an hour or so each week creating your own snack packs. You'll have more variety, spend less money, and will always have something to throw into your briefcase, purse, pocket, or backpack.

Non-Dieting Family Members

One of the difficulties of dieting for many parents is that the rest of the family doesn't want to diet with them. This leaves them having to choose between cooking a separate meal for themselves or blowing their diet at dinnertime. To help sidestep this issue, make lunch your main meal. This is actually the way most Mediterranean people eat, leaving dinner as a lighter meal.

By making lunch your main meal and having a healthful snack shortly before dinner, you can prepare vegetables and other sides for the family that are Mediterranean friendly and skip any entrees that aren't on your diet.

Exercise Naturally

In addition to the dietary changes you'll be making, you'll receive the most benefit from the Mediterranean diet if you also follow its philosophy of enjoying your life and your health by building exercise into your daily activities and lowering your stress. These strategies will also help you maximize weight loss and build a stronger, healthier body.

Many Americans were resentful and a bit envious a few years ago when there was a great deal of publicity about the fact that regimented exercise isn't very common in Europe and the Mediterranean, and yet overweight and obese people are far more rare there than they are here.

The fact is that in Europe and the Mediterranean, exercise is built into daily life in such a way that people stay fit while doing other things they enjoy. The exercise is almost a by-product of enjoying the fresh air, friends, and family.

Rather than getting peeved over it, get excited! This practice will work for you, too. Here are some ways to get in exercise without feeling like you're working out.

- **Dance!** Do it alone, with your toddler, or with your romantic partner. Throw on some music and just have fun. Try new dance styles, such as belly dancing, hula, or Latin dance.
- **Play!** Chances are, you need to exercise but you don't want to give up time with your kids. Combine the two. Have a game of kickball or volleyball, go bike riding, play tag or hide and seek, or make an after-dinner walk a way to spend quality time with your child.
- **Get outside!** There are a lot of outdoor activities that most people don't consider exercise, even though they pack a fitness wallop. Try hiking, surfing, kayaking, skating, or horseback riding. They all work your body and get you outside to enjoy great weather and fresh, reviving air.

Lower Stress to Help Burn Body Fat

You've probably heard about the connection between stress, the stress hormone cortisol, and belly fat. There is plenty of well-respected research that shows that even the stress of daily life can stimulate the release of cortisol into your bloodstream, and that cortisol's main directive is to store belly fat. This natural response to stress may have been useful back when you were running from a stampede of mastodon, but now . . . not so much.

This connection between stress and belly fat may be part of the reason that the people of the Mediterranean have fewer issues with obesity and abdominal fat. They eat more healthfully, and they live more healthfully when it comes to stress. Their lives are generally not as hurried, their days not as full.

Here are a number of things you can do to reduce the effects of stress on your body and reduce the amount of cortisol released into your bloodstream.

- **Get adequate sleep.** Studies have shown that people who sleep less than six hours a night have significantly higher blood cortisol levels and abdominal fat.
- **Enjoy recreation time.** Spend at least fifteen minutes a day doing something just for you. That could mean a walk in the garden, a bubble bath, or relaxing with a soothing CD.
- **Laugh.** Do it often and do it for real. If you need help, rent a comedy video or call your wittiest friend.
- **Take vitamin C.** Vitamin C is depleted constantly, especially by stress. This enormously important vitamin is essential for cell building, and it also stimulates the production of carnitine, which is used to transport stored fat to where it can be metabolized. In other words, once you reduce stress to reduce cortisol, the carnitine will take that belly fat you don't need anymore to where it can be used for energy. Talk about a win-win.

Gauging Your Success

Even if your main objective in following the Mediterranean diet is to lose weight, be careful of placing too much emphasis on the numbers on the scale. Here are some other very important ways to measure your success, in addition to pounds lost.

- **Inches lost.** If you're exercising regularly, you'll start building muscle. Muscle weighs more than fat but takes up much less space. Inches lost can be a much more accurate indicator of how you're doing.
- **How your clothes fit.** Even if you don't take your measurements regularly, pay attention to how your clothes are fitting. If your waistband no longer strangles you and you have more room in your jeans, you're doing well.
- **Your energy level.** Eating healthful, balanced meals and ditching unhealthful ones will give you a boost of energy that will help you live more actively and fully.
- **Your physical exams.** Lower cholesterol levels, lower heart rate and blood pressure, and fewer indicators of prediabetes are some of the benefits reaped by many people who follow the Mediterranean diet. If your lab tests, blood work, and doctor say you're looking good, you're looking good.

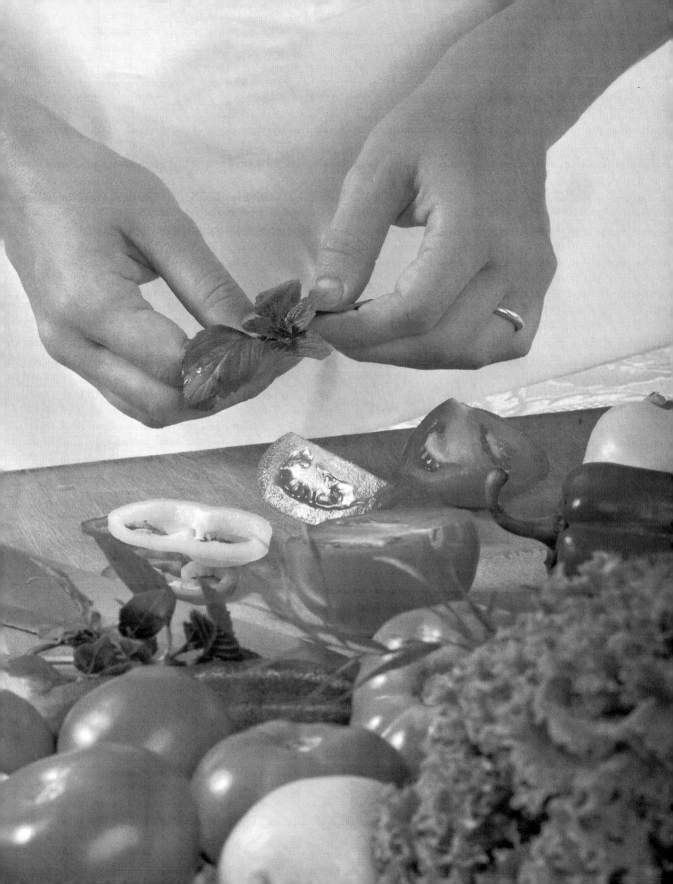

(5)

COOKING METHODS THAT MAKE A DIFFERENCE

Almost as important as the foods you choose are the methods you use to cook them. The cooking methods favored by the Mediterranean people maximize flavor and freshness without adding unnecessary fats and calories.

As you might imagine, deep-fried foods are out. Deep frying generally involves fats such as vegetable or peanut oils, which shouldn't be in your house if you're going for good health. Don't worry; you have loads of other options.

Roasting, baking, broiling, sautéing, grilling, and steaming are all great methods to cook your food beautifully and healthfully. Roasting and grilling are the favorite means by which the Mediterranean people prepare most meats, fish, and vegetables. Steaming is another option for veggies and fish, but roasting brings out a great deal of flavor that you'll miss with steaming.

Stews and soups are also popular choices, and they allow busy cooks to prepare hearty, delicious meals with very little time spent in the kitchen.

Avoid boiling or simmering poultry and vegetables unless you'll be using the broth (strained of any fats) for stock, soup, or a sauce. Most nutrients and flavor are lost in the water, and limp, watery veggies are what makes kids (and adults) think they're so boring.

Sautéing is great for foods that require minimal cooking time, such as mushrooms, leafy vegetables and some shellfish. The high heat and quick cooking locks in color and flavor.

The Fast Way to Fabulous Veggies

Here's a simple way to roast most any vegetable, from asparagus to zucchini to carrots:

Trim or peel the veggies as needed. Line a baking sheet or dish with foil and add a quarter-sized portion of olive oil. Dump in the veggies and mix them with your clean hands until they are well coated (rub the oil onto the back of your hands before rinsing for an added moisturizing effect!). Add salt, pepper, and any other seasonings to the vegetables. Roast 10–30 minutes (depending on the vegetable and the size of the pieces), place into a serving dish or your plate, and throw away the foil.

You'll have amazingly sweet, perfectly caramelized veggies, younger, softer hands, and no pan to wash. For a busy cook, it doesn't get much better than that.

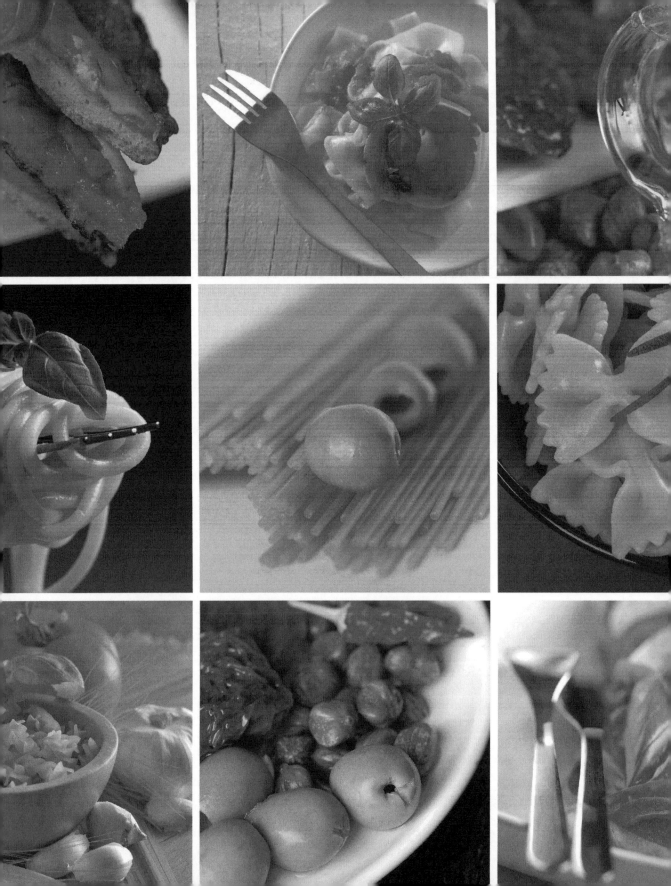

SECTION TWO

Mediterranean Diet Recipes

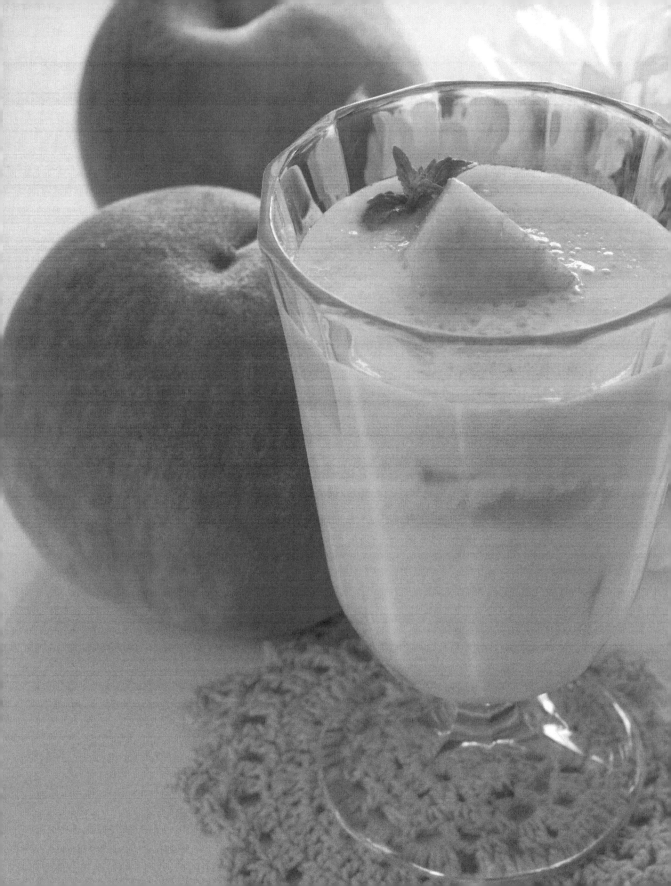

BREAKFAST

Everyone has heard the admonition that breakfast is the most important meal of the day. Dieters have been hearing that a lot; as people learn more about how the metabolism works, they find that breakfast is even more important than they already thought.

Your metabolism is at its slowest when you wake up in the morning. Your body's energy has been directed toward digestion and no new fuel has entered your system in several hours, which slows the metabolism even more. To rev up your metabolism, you need to eat as soon after waking as you can (or can stand). If you skip breakfast, you'll have a hard time sticking to any diet, as you follow your body's cravings for carbs and sugar to give it the boost it needs.

Some Helpful Meal Ideas

That being said, there are plenty of great options for your morning meal.

If you don't care for most traditional breakfast foods such as cereal or eggs, let go of your traditional view of breakfast. Any combination of protein, fiber, and carbs will do. Have some cheese, fruit, and crusty bread, or even a cup of soup leftover from last night.

If you do have the time and inclination to eat breakfast, try to include protein, such as eggs or Greek yogurt, as well as fiber-rich grains (multi-grain cereals and whole-grain toast) and fruits.

If time is at a premium in the mornings, try a smoothie. You can pack quite a bit of nutrition into a smoothie and the possibilities are endless. Even though the diet advocates mindful, peaceful eating, sipping a smoothie while you get the kids off to school or drive your commute is better than skipping your morning meal.

Spinach, Mushroom, and Ricotta Breakfast Sandwich

This open-faced sandwich is a new way to enjoy the traditional Florentine ingredients of spinach and cheese, and makes a great brunch entrée. You can make the ricotta filling up to two days ahead to save time in the morning.

- 2 teaspoons olive oil
- 1 medium yellow onion, finely chopped
- 1 clove garlic, crushed
- 1/2 cup sliced white mushrooms
- 2 cups spinach leaves
- 1/2 teaspoon fresh oregano
- 1/2 teaspoon sea salt
- 1/2 teaspoon white pepper
- 1 cup part-skim ricotta cheese, room temperature
- 4 slices whole-grain bread, toasted

In a medium-sized heavy skillet, heat the olive oil over medium heat.

Add the onion and garlic, and sauté, stirring frequently, for about 5 minutes or until onion is just translucent.

Add the mushrooms and cook for 2 minutes, then add the spinach and sauté for another 5 minutes. Meanwhile, preheat the broiler.

Season the vegetable mixture with the oregano, sea salt, and white pepper, and stir in the ricotta cheese, mixing well.

Place the toast onto a baking sheet lined with foil. Divide the mixture between the 4 slices.

Broil 3 inches from heat, just until the cheese begins to bubble. To serve, place one slice onto each plate and cut in half diagonally. Serve with fresh fruit.

Serves 4.

Almond Latte Smoothie

For coffee lovers, it's easier to go without breakfast than to go without coffee. Since you shouldn't skip breakfast, this chilly drink will help you have both your morning meal and your morning coffee, no matter how rushed you are. The egg whites are pasteurized, so no worries about including them.

- 1/2 cup brewed espresso, room temperature
- 1 1/2 cups vanilla almond milk
- Sweetener, to taste
- 2 packaged egg whites
- 8–10 ice cubes

In a blender, combine the espresso, almond milk, and sweetener, and blend until well mixed.

Add the egg whites and ice cubes and blend until thick and smooth. Drink immediately.

Serves 2.

Apple-Feta-Walnut Breakfast Tortilla

If you enjoy apple pie with cheddar cheese, try this breakfast dish. It's a great breakfast for lazy weekends and cool mornings. The apple filling can be doubled up and prepared up to a week ahead.

- 6 firm apples, such as Gala, peeled and cored
- 1 teaspoon cinnamon
- 1/4 teaspoon sea salt
- 1 teaspoon olive oil
- 2 teaspoons light brown sugar
- 1/4 cup chopped walnuts
- 4 (6-inch) whole-grain, whole-wheat tortillas
- 1 cup crumbled feta cheese

Preheat oven to 400 degrees.

Slice the apples about 1/4-inch thick and sprinkle with the cinnamon and sea salt.

Heat the olive oil in a medium-sized heavy saucepan over medium-high heat.

Add the apple slices in a single layer and sauté for about 5 minutes before turning each slice over. Carefully drain the oil and water from the apples.

Sprinkle the apples with the brown sugar and add the walnuts to the pan. Cook for another 2–4 minutes, until the apples begin to caramelize and the sugar is melted. Remove from heat.

Line a baking sheet with aluminum foil and place the tortillas on the baking sheet. Divide the apple filling between them and top with the crumbled feta cheese.

Bake for 5–7 minutes or until apples are browned and the cheese is mostly melted.

To serve, cut each tortilla into four wedges. Serve alongside scrambled eggs or an omelet.

Serves 4.

Honey and Avocado Smoothie

Avocados are loaded with heart-healthful monounsaturated fats and will definitely fill you up in the morning. While common in savory dishes in the Americas, in other parts of the world avocados are used in sweet drinks and desserts.

- 1 1/2 cups milk of your choice
- 1 large avocado

- 2 tablespoons honey

Add all ingredients to your blender and blend until smooth and creamy.

Serve immediately and enjoy!

Serves 2.

Apple and Tahini Toast

Tahini is a paste made from sesame seeds, and is high in vitamins B1, B2, B3, B5, and B15. Similar to peanut butter, it's often found in dips such as hummus. In some countries, it is commonly served for breakfast with toast.

- 2 tablespoons tahini
- 2 slices whole-wheat bread, toasted
- 1 small apple of your choice, cored and thinly sliced
- 1 teaspoon honey

Spread the tahini on the toasted bread.

Lay the apples on the bread and drizzle with honey.

Serve immediately.

Serves 1.

Peach and Walnut Breakfast Salad

Ripe fruit served in season is a hallmark of Mediterranean cuisine. This dish is light and fresh but feels just a little bit like dessert. If you prefer, substitute apples for the pears. Serve with whole-grain toast for a complete breakfast.

- 1/2 cup low-fat or nonfat cottage cheese, room temperature
- 1 ripe peach, pitted and sliced
- 1/4 cup chopped walnuts, toasted
- 1 teaspoon honey
- 1 tablespoon chopped fresh mint
- Zest of 1 lemon

Put the cottage cheese in a small bowl, and top with the peach slices and walnuts.

Drizzle with the honey, then top with the fresh mint and a pinch of lemon zest.

Serve with a spoon.

Serves 1.

Peachy Green Smoothie

You'll get many servings of fruits and vegetables in one delicious drink with this smoothie. It's perfect for days when cooking for yourself is a challenge. Don't forget to use Greek yogurt.

- 1 cup almond milk
- 3 cups kale or spinach
- 1 banana, peeled
- 1 orange, peeled
- 1 small green apple
- 1 cup frozen peaches
- 1/4 cup vanilla Greek yogurt

Put the ingredients in a blender in the order listed and blend on high until smooth.

Serve and enjoy.

Serves 2.

Cinnamon Bulgur with Berries

Bulgur is easy to cook and full of fiber, but it is also low in fat and calories. While commonly used in more savory dishes, it makes a lovely hot breakfast, especially when paired with cinnamon and berries. Serve this cereal dish instead of oatmeal on a chilly morning.

- 1/2 cup medium-grain bulgur wheat
- 1 cup water
- Pinch sea salt
- 1/4 cup milk

- 1 teaspoon pure vanilla extract
- 1/4 teaspoon ground cinnamon
- 1 cup fresh berries of your choice

Put the bulgur in a medium saucepan with the water and sea salt, and bring to a boil.

Cover, remove from heat, and let stand for 10 minutes until water is absorbed.

Stir in the milk, vanilla, and cinnamon until fully incorporated.

Divide between 2 bowls and top with the fresh berries to serve.

Serves 2.

Savory Breakfast Oats

This savory hot cereal combines the fiber of oats with the juicy, sunny flavors common in Turkey, Greece, and Israel. Meanwhile, the herbs and pepper add a little zip.

- 1/2 cup steel-cut oats
- 1 cup water
- 1 large tomato, chopped
- 1 medium cucumber, chopped
- 1 tablespoon olive oil
- Freshly grated low-fat Parmesan cheese
- Flat-leaf parsley or mint, chopped, for garnish
- Sea salt and freshly ground pepper, to taste

Put the oats and 1 cup of water in a medium saucepan and bring to a boil on high heat.

Stir continuously until water is absorbed, about 15 minutes.

To serve, divide the oatmeal between 2 bowls and top with the tomatoes and cucumber.

Drizzle with olive oil, then top with the Parmesan cheese and parsley or mint.

Season to taste.

Serve immediately.

Serves 2.

Fresh Veggie Frittata

You can use whatever ingredients you have for this recipe—grilled or roasted vegetables add great depth of flavor, as well as nutrition.

- 3 large eggs
- 1 teaspoon almond milk
- 1 tablespoon olive oil
- 1 handful baby spinach leaves
- 1/2 baby eggplant, peeled and diced
- 1/4 small red bell pepper, chopped
- Sea salt and freshly ground pepper, to taste
- 1 ounce crumbled goat cheese

Preheat the broiler.

Beat the eggs with the almond milk until just combined.

Heat a small nonstick, broiler-proof skillet over medium-high heat. Add the olive oil, followed by the eggs.

Spread the spinach on top of the egg mixture in an even layer and top with the rest of the veggies.

Reduce heat to medium and season with sea salt and freshly ground pepper to taste. Allow the eggs and vegetables to cook 3–5 minutes until the bottom half of the eggs are firm and vegetables are tender.

Top with the crumbled goat cheese and place on middle rack under the broiler, and then cook another 3–5 minutes until the eggs are firm in the middle and the cheese has melted.

Slice into wedges and serve immediately.

Serves 1.

Scrambled Eggs with Feta and Olives

The Mediterranean is the birthplace of olives, and Spain the largest producer. Skip bland canned olives, which are cured using lye. Choose French, Italian, or Greek varieties available at olive bars, instead.

- 4 large eggs
- 1 tablespoon milk
- Sea salt, to taste
- 1 tablespoon olive oil
- 1/4 cup crumbled feta cheese
- 10 Kalamata olives, pitted and sliced
- Freshly ground pepper, to taste
- Small bunch fresh mint, chopped

Beat the eggs with a fork or wire whisk until just combined.

Add the milk and a pinch of sea salt.

Heat a medium nonstick skillet over medium-high heat and add the olive oil.

Add the eggs and stir constantly, until they just begin to curd and firm up.

Add the feta cheese and olives, and stir until evenly combined.

Season with sea salt and freshly ground pepper to taste. Use a light hand with the salt, because the olives and feta are very salty.

Divide between 2 plates and garnish with the fresh chopped mint. Serve immediately.

Serves 2.

Garlic Scrambled Eggs with Basil

This version of scrambled eggs is anything but bland. Basil and garlic add Mediterranean flavor to this breakfast staple. Serve with whole-grain toast or a fruit and nut muffin.

- 4 large eggs
- 2 tablespoons finely chopped fresh basil
- 2 tablespoons grated Gruyère cheese
- 1 tablespoon cream
- 1 tablespoon olive oil
- 2 cloves garlic, minced
- Sea salt and freshly ground pepper, to taste

In a large bowl, beat together the eggs, basil, cheese, and cream with a whisk until just combined.

Heat the oil in a large, heavy nonstick skillet over medium-low heat. Add the garlic and cook until golden, about 1 minute.

Pour the egg mixture into the skillet over the garlic. Work the eggs continuously and cook until fluffy and soft.

Season with sea salt and freshly ground pepper to taste.

Divide between 2 plates and serve immediately.

Serves 2.

Spanish Tuna Tortilla with Roasted Peppers

A tortilla is a popular Spanish egg dish, similar to an omelet, but made with potatoes. While often served as a small plate or "tapa" at bars, it also makes a great breakfast dish.

- 6 large eggs
- 1/4 cup olive oil
- 2 small Russet potatoes, diced
- 1 small onion, chopped
- 1 roasted red bell pepper, sliced
- 1 (7-ounce) can tuna packed in water, drained well and flaked
- 2 plum tomatoes, seeded and diced
- 1 teaspoon dried tarragon

Preheat the broiler on high.

Crack the eggs in a large bowl and whisk them together until just combined.

Heat the olive oil in a large, oven-safe, nonstick or cast-iron skillet over medium-low heat.

Add the potatoes and cook until slightly soft, about 7 minutes.

Add the onion and the peppers and cook until soft, 3–5 minutes.

Add the tuna, tomatoes, and tarragon to the skillet and stir to combine, then add the eggs.

Cook for 7–10 minutes until the eggs are bubbling from the bottom and the bottom is slightly brown.

Place the skillet into the oven on 1 of the first 2 racks, and cook until the middle is set and the top is slightly brown.

Slice into wedges and serve warm or at room temperature.

Serves 4.

Greek Eggs and Potatoes

Eggs get a nutritional and flavor boost from fresh tomatoes, herbs, and garlic. Leave the peel on potatoes for more fiber and texture. This dish can be served family-style at the table, if you prefer.

- 3 medium tomatoes, seeded and coarsely chopped
- 2 tablespoons fresh chopped basil
- 1 garlic clove, minced
- 2 tablespoons plus 1/2 cup olive oil, divided
- Sea salt and freshly ground pepper, to taste
- 3 large russet potatoes
- 4 large eggs
- 1 teaspoon fresh oregano, chopped

Put tomatoes in a food processor and puree them, skins and all.

Add the basil, garlic, 2 tablespoons olive oil, sea salt, and freshly ground pepper, and pulse to combine.

Put the mixture in a large skillet over low heat and cook, covered, for 20–25 minutes, or until the sauce has thickened and is bubbly.

Meanwhile, dice the potatoes into small cubes. Put 1/2 cup olive oil in a nonstick skillet over medium-low heat.

Fry the potatoes for 5 minutes until crisp and browned on the outside, then cover and reduce heat to low. Steam potatoes until done.

Carefully crack the eggs into the tomato sauce. Cook over low heat until the eggs are set in the sauce, about 6 minutes.

Remove the potatoes from the pan and drain them on paper towels, then place them in a bowl.

Sprinkle with sea salt and freshly ground pepper to taste and top with the oregano.

Carefully remove the eggs with a slotted spoon and place them on a plate with the potatoes. Spoon sauce over the top and serve.

Serves 2.

Spiced Scrambled Eggs

You can enjoy whole eggs up to four times a week on the Mediterranean diet. Spicy additions like the Fresno or jalapeño peppers included here not only add flavor but can help you feel full faster. Enjoy with sliced tomatoes and whole-wheat toast.

- 2 tablespoons olive oil
- 1 small red onion, chopped
- 1 medium green pepper, cored, seeded, and finely chopped
- 1 red Fresno or jalapeño chili pepper, seeded and cut into thin strips
- 3 medium tomatoes, chopped
- Sea salt and freshly ground pepper, to taste
- 1 tablespoon ground cumin
- 1 teaspoon ground coriander
- 4 large eggs, lightly beaten

Heat the olive oil in a large, heavy skillet over medium heat.

Add the onion and cook until soft and translucent, 6–7 minutes.

Add the peppers and continue to cook until soft, another 4–5 minutes.

Add in the tomatoes and season to taste.

Stir in the cumin and coriander.

Simmer for 10 minutes over medium-low heat.

Add the eggs, stirring them into the mixture to distribute.

Cover the skillet and cook until the eggs are set but still fluffy and tender, about 5–6 minutes more.

Divide between 4 plates and serve immediately.

Serves 4.

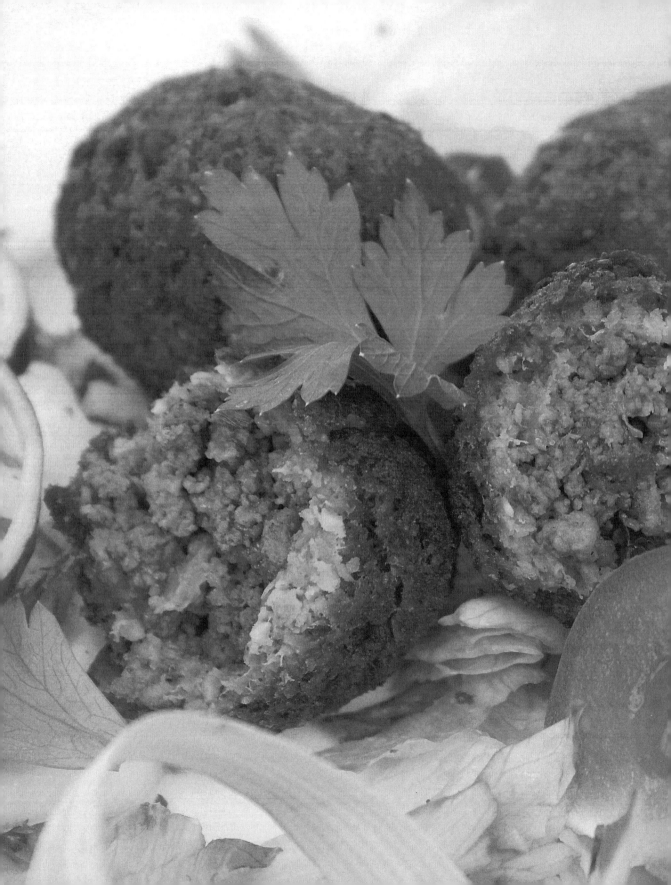

LUNCH

It's very easy to fail to eat a healthful lunch, especially one that adheres to the Mediterranean diet principles. People are often too rushed and too starved to bother with having a delicious, healthful lunch.

If you're eating your breakfast and having frequent snacks, you should be feeling satisfied enough to avoid those afternoon binges on deli food or drive-through lunches. The key then is to have meals available or accessible that follow your plan.

As stated earlier, it's important to eat intentionally and consciously on the Mediterranean diet. Slowing down, focusing on what you're eating, and really enjoying it is important.

If at all possible, schedule time to enjoy your lunch in a nice atmosphere, whether you're alone or with coworkers and friends. If you're at work, try skipping the cafeteria, break room, or kitchen and head outside to a patio or park. If you're at home, put a flower on your table, put on some nice music, and eat on one of your prettiest plates.

Meal Ideas for Lunch

If you're at home during the lunch hour or when you're home on weekends, you have any and all meal options open to you. However, if you're at work or out with friends at a favorite restaurant, you might feel a bit more challenged. Here are some ideas to help.

At Work

Purchase an inexpensive, insulated lunch bag and some small containers to take a healthful lunch and some snacks to work. Get in the habit of filling it every night, and you'll be less likely to dash out the door empty-handed and end up at the drive-through.

Some good meal ideas are a clear soup, such as barley, vegetable, minestrone, or miso, accompanied by a small sandwich on whole grain bread or a roll. Salads are also a great option. Load up on the veggies (and try fruits in your salads, as well), and pack the dressing in a separate container.

You can make two meals in one by cooking an extra serving or two of every healthful, Mediterranean dinner, then freeze it in portion-sized containers for later lunches.

In just a couple of weeks, you'll have quite a stockpile of your own frozen entrees to choose from. They'll be great for lunch and handy for those evenings when you forgot to thaw the chicken.

At a Restaurant

If you go out to lunch frequently, you may face quite a few temptations and challenges, but sticking to the Mediterranean diet is still very doable.

Japanese, Thai, vegetarian, seafood, Greek, and some American restaurants can be great places to eat lunch on the Mediterranean diet. Mexican, buffet, Chinese, and (ironically) many Italian restaurants can be very challenging and aren't your best bet.

Drink a bottle or glass of water and munch an apple or a handful of nuts and dried fruit about an hour before lunch. This will keep you from falling face first into the breadbasket later. In fact, if possible, ask the server not to bring bread at all, unless the restaurant serves whole-grain artisan breads. If your dining companions want bread, just let them know that you need to skip it and hopefully they won't try to tempt or tease you into having some. If they do, you may want to look for different lunch companions!

Opt for a healthful salad with a vinaigrette or oil and vinegar dressing and without croutons (usually deep-fried), Parmesan (too much fat and salt), or bacon bits (too much bacon!).

Again, clear soups are a great way to get a hearty meal and still stick with the program.

Fish broiled or baked without butter and shrimp are also great, if you feel the need for a full entrée.

White Bean, Cherry Tomato, and Kale Soup

White beans and kale are typical of Tuscany. This soup is as inexpensive as it is filling and nutritious. If you want to make this completely vegetarian, substitute vegetable stock.

- 2 tablespoons olive oil
- 1 small onion, chopped
- 2 cloves garlic, minced
- 1 bunch kale, torn into bite-sized pieces
- 6 cups chicken or vegetable broth
- 2 pints cherry tomatoes, halved
- 2 cans white beans of your choice, drained and rinsed
- Sea salt and freshly ground pepper, to taste
- Freshly grated low-fat Parmesan cheese

Heat the olive oil in a large soup pot or Dutch oven over medium heat.

Add the onions and cook for 5 minutes, or until soft and translucent.

Add the garlic and cook for 1 more minute.

Add the kale and stir until well coated with the olive oil.

Add the broth and bring to boil on high heat.

Reduce heat to low, and simmer for 15 minutes, until kale is softened.

Add the tomatoes and beans, and simmer for 5 more minutes.

Season with sea salt and freshly ground pepper to taste.

To serve, ladle into bowls, and sprinkle with Parmesan cheese.

Serves 4.

Shrimp Soup with Leeks and Fennel

The Provençal flavors of leeks, fennel, garlic, and shrimp are featured in this elegant soup. Soup like this is low in calories yet filling, and provides several servings of vegetables. You can substitute scallops for the shrimp, if you prefer.

- 2 tablespoons olive oil
- 3 stalks celery, chopped
- 1 leek, both whites and light green parts, sliced
- 1 medium fennel bulb, chopped
- 1 clove garlic, minced
- Sea salt and freshly ground pepper, to taste
- 1 tablespoon fennel seeds
- 4 cups vegetable or chicken broth
- 1 pound medium shrimp, peeled and deveined
- 2 tablespoons light cream
- Juice of 1 lemon

Heat the oil in a large Dutch oven over medium heat.

Add the celery, leek, and fennel, and cook for about 15 minutes, until vegetables are browned and very soft.

Add the garlic and season with sea salt and freshly ground pepper to taste. Add the fennel seed and stir. Add the broth and bring to a boil, then reduce to a simmer and cook about 20 more minutes.

Add the shrimp to the soup and cook until just pink, about 3 minutes.

Add the cream and lemon juice, and serve immediately.

Serves 6.

Turkish Lentil Soup

Lentil soup is one of the most inexpensive, nutritious foods you can make. If you can't find green lentils, substitute brown. This Turkish-inspired recipe is vegetarian, but feel free to add shredded ham or chicken for a more robust dish.

- 2 tablespoons olive oil
- 1 small onion, diced
- 2 tablespoons flour
- 4 cups water or chicken stock
- 1 1/2 cups green lentils
- 1 carrot, peeled and diced
- 1/2 teaspoon dried thyme
- 1 teaspoon sea salt
- 1/2 teaspoon freshly ground pepper

Heat the olive oil in a large stockpot on medium-high heat.

Sauté the onions just until tender and translucent. Whisk in the flour, stirring for 30 seconds until thickened into a paste.

Slowly whisk in the water or chicken stock 1/4 cup at a time, and bring to a boil, stirring frequently.

Add the lentils, carrot, and seasonings. Cover and simmer for 1 hour, or until lentils are tender.

Serves 6.

Riviera Tuna Salad

Humble canned tuna becomes something special in this healthful, main-dish salad, while garbanzo beans add fiber and protein.

- 1/4 cup olive oil
- 1/4 cup balsamic vinegar
- 1/2 teaspoon minced garlic
- 1/4 teaspoon dried oregano
- Sea salt and freshly ground pepper, to taste
- 2 tablespoons capers, drained
- 4–6 cups baby greens
- 1 (6-ounce) can solid white albacore tuna, drained
- 1 cup canned garbanzo beans, rinsed and drained
- 1/4 cup low-salt olives, pitted and quartered
- 2 Roma tomatoes, chopped

To make the vinaigrette, whisk together the olive oil, balsamic vinegar, garlic, oregano, sea salt, and pepper until emulsified. Stir in the capers.

Refrigerate for up to 6 hours before serving.

Place the baby greens in a salad bowl or on individual plates, and top with the tuna, beans, olives, and tomatoes.

Drizzle the vinaigrette over all, and serve immediately.

Serves 4.

Warm Fennel, Cherry Tomato, and Spinach Salad

Slightly wilted spinach contrasts nicely with the crunchy fennel in this salad that can serve as a side dish or even a light lunch.

- 4 tablespoons chicken broth
- 4 cups baby spinach leaves
- 10 cherry tomatoes, halved
- Sea salt and freshly ground pepper, to taste

- 1 fennel bulb, sliced
- 1/4 cup olive oil
- Juice of 2 lemons

In a large sauté pan, heat the chicken broth over medium heat. Add the spinach and tomatoes and toss until spinach is wilted. Season with sea salt and freshly ground pepper to taste.

Remove from heat and toss fennel slices in with the spinach and tomatoes. Let the fennel warm in the pan, and then transfer to a large bowl.

Drizzle with the olive oil and lemon juice, and serve immediately.

Serves 2.

Four-Bean Salad

Beans are a staple in many parts of the Mediterranean. High in fiber, beans are also versatile and can be eaten hot or cold, in salads or soups. Use dried beans for the best flavor, but keep canned beans on hand as a convenient option.

- 1/2 cup white beans, cooked
- 1/2 cup black-eyed peas, cooked
- 1/2 cup fava beans, cooked
- 1/2 cup lima beans, cooked
- 1 red bell pepper, diced
- 1 small bunch flat-leaf parsley, chopped
- 2 tablespoons olive oil
- 1 teaspoon ground cumin
- Juice of 1 lemon
- Sea salt and freshly ground pepper, to taste

You can cook the beans a day or two in advance to speed up the preparation of this dish.

Combine all ingredients in a large bowl and mix well.

Season to taste.

Allow to sit for 30 minutes, so the flavors can come together before serving.

Serves 4.

Beef Gyros

Classic Greek gyros are often made from lamb, but these beef gyros are easy and delicious. Using pita bread minimizes the carbohydrates in this sandwich. You could also make this with leftover lean roast beef.

For the tzatziki:
- 2 cups Greek yogurt
- 3 tablespoons lemon juice
- 4 cloves garlic, minced
- 1 medium cucumber, peeled, seeded, and grated
- 1/2 teaspoon cumin
- 4–5 mint leaves, chopped
- Sea salt and freshly ground pepper, to taste

For the marinade:
- 1/2 onion, quartered
- 1/4 cup water
- 3 cloves garlic
- 2 tablespoons sugar
- 1 teaspoon prepared mustard
- 1 teaspoon freshly ground pepper
- 1 tablespoon olive oil
- 1/2 teaspoon ground ginger
- 1/2 teaspoon cayenne pepper

For the filling:
- 1 1/2 pounds sirloin tip roast cut into 1-inch strips
- 1 package pita bread
- 1 head romaine, chopped into ribbons
- 2 tomatoes, chopped
- 1 red onion, thinly sliced

Make the tzatziki:

Stir together the yogurt, lemon juice, garlic, cucumber, cumin, and mint in a small bowl until smooth.

Season with sea salt and freshly ground pepper to taste.

Make the marinade:

Combine all the marinade ingredients in a food processor and process until smooth.

Pour the marinade into a plastic bag or shallow dish.

Make the filling:

Place the beef in the marinade and refrigerate for at least 4 hours, or overnight. Drain.

Grill meat in a grill basket over medium-high heat for 6–8 minutes, or until cooked through. Remove from the heat.

Warm pita bread on the grill, or in a toaster oven.

Place some of the cooked meat inside the pita. Top with the lettuce, tomato, red onion, and cucumber sauce.

Serve the gyros with a green salad or roasted potatoes.

Serves 6.

Dolmades

Dolmades are stuffed grape leaves, a popular appetizer in Greece, where they are usually served with tzatziki, a cucumber yogurt sauce. This complex vegetarian version features rice, herbs, buttery pine nuts, sweet raisins, and tangy lemon.

- 1 tablespoon olive oil
- 3 shallots, chopped
- 2 cloves garlic, minced
- 3/4 cup short-grain rice
- 1/4 cup gold raisins
- 1/4 cup pine nuts, toasted
- Juice of 1 lemon
- Sea salt and freshly ground pepper, to taste
- 2/3 cup water
- 4 green onions, chopped
- 1 small bunch mint leaves, finely chopped
- 1 small bunch flat-leaf parsley, chopped
- 20 preserved grape leaves

Heat the olive oil in large skillet over medium heat.

Add the shallots and garlic, and sauté for 5 minutes. Add the rice, golden raisins, pine nuts, and lemon juice. Season with sea salt and freshly ground pepper.

Add 2/3 cup water, bring to a boil, and cover. Reduce heat and simmer for 20 minutes. Turn off heat and allow rice to cool.

Add the green onions and herbs to the rice filling and mix well.

Rinse the grape leaves in water and stuff each leaf with about 1 tablespoon of the filling.

Roll tightly and place each in a steamer, seam side down.

Steam for about 10 minutes, until leaves are tender.

Serve warm.

Makes 20.

Roasted Eggplant Dip with Spicy Yogurt Sauce and Homemade Pita Chips

Roasting eggplant softens it and adds a smoky flavor. This dip is reminiscent of Lebanese baba ghanoush, and the yogurt dip is much like Greek tzatziki. For added nutrition, include raw vegetables with the pita chips for dipping.

For the eggplant dip:

- 2 large eggplants
- Pinch of sea salt
- Juice of 2 lemons
- 2 bell peppers, diced
- 2 roasted red peppers, diced
- 2 cups diced tomatoes
- 20 yellow or red cherry tomatoes
- 5 cloves garlic, minced
- 1/2 cup chopped flat-leaf parsley
- 1/4 cup chives, chopped
- 3 basil leaves, slivered
- 1 tablespoon olive oil
- Sea salt and freshly ground pepper, to taste

For the yogurt sauce:

- 1 cup Greek yogurt
- 1/2 cucumber, grated
- 2 tablespoons fresh dill, chopped
- 1 clove garlic, minced
- 1 jalapeño, chopped
- Sea salt and freshly ground pepper, to taste

For the pita chips:

- 4 whole-wheat pitas, each cut into 12 triangles
- 2 tablespoons olive oil
- 1 teaspoon sesame seeds
- Sea salt and freshly ground pepper, to taste

Make the eggplant dip:

Preheat oven to 450 degrees.

Salt both sides of the sliced eggplant, and let sit for 20 minutes to draw out the bitter juices. Rinse the eggplant and pat dry with a paper towel.

Roast eggplants until they fall, about 35 minutes. Cool and cut open, scooping out the flesh. Throw away skins. Drizzle eggplant with lemon juice and put into a strainer, then squeeze out moisture.

Chop and mix with peppers, tomato, garlic, herbs, and olive oil.

Season with sea salt and freshly ground pepper.

Make the yogurt sauce:

Mix yogurt, cucumber, dill, garlic, and jalapeño. Season with sea salt and freshly ground pepper.

Make the pita chips:

Reduce oven temp to 350 degrees.

Lay wedges on baking sheet, then drizzle with olive oil, sprinkle with sesame seeds, sea salt, and freshly ground pepper.

Bake for 10–15 minutes until crisp.

Serve the pita chips with the yogurt sauce and roasted eggplant.

Serves 8.

Falafel

Falafel is a traditional Middle Eastern food thought to have originated in Egypt, but it is considered the national dish of Israel. It is made from chickpeas, which are a good source of fiber and protein. Add any vegetables you'd like to the finished sandwich, such as cucumbers or shredded lettuce.

For the tahini sauce:

- 1/2 cup tahini sauce
- 1/4 cup flat-leaf parsley, finely chopped
- 2 tablespoons lemon juice
- 2 cloves garlic, minced
- 1/2 cup cold water, as needed

For the falafel:

- 1 cup dried chickpeas, soaked overnight
- 1 large onion, chopped
- 1/4 cup flat-leaf parsley, chopped
- 1/4 cup cilantro, chopped

- 4 cloves garlic, peeled
- 1 teaspoon sea salt
- 1 teaspoon cumin
- 1/2 teaspoon chili flakes
- 1 1/2 teaspoons baking soda, dissolved in 1 teaspoon water
- 4–6 tablespoons flour
- 2 cups peanut oil
- 1 tomato, chopped
- 1 bell pepper, chopped
- 4 pita rounds

Make the tahini sauce:

Whisk the tahini, parsley, lemon juice, and garlic together until creamy. Add up to 1/2 cup cold water as needed to thin the sauce and make it smooth and creamy.

Cover and refrigerate while you make the falafel.

Make the falafel:

Drain the chickpeas and add them to a large food processor with the onion, parsley, cilantro, garlic, sea salt, cumin, and chili flakes.

Process until well mixed but not pureed, then add the baking soda and flour, and pulse until you have a dough. (The dough should hold together and not stick to your hands. Add flour as needed to keep dough from being too tacky.)

Cover dough in a large bowl and refrigerate for several hours.

Form the dough into small balls the size of walnuts.

Heat 3 inches of oil to 375 degrees in a large pot. Fry one ball and see if it holds together. If the ball falls apart, add more flour to the dough.

Then fry the chickpea balls 6 at a time, turning to make sure they are golden brown on all sides, and drain on a paper towel.

Stuff pitas with falafel balls, garnish with tomatoes and bell peppers, and drizzle with tahini sauce.

Serves 4.

Italian Breaded Shrimp Stuffed with Couscous

Couscous and shrimp have one thing in common (besides being delicious): they are both super fast to cook. Sundried tomatoes and pesto add Italian flavor to this festive dish. Use the largest shrimp you can find to make the stuffing easy.

- 1 cup vegetable stock
- 1/2 cup whole-wheat couscous
- 12 extra-large shrimp, peeled and deveined
- 1 egg, beaten
- 1/4 cup Italian-seasoned breadcrumbs

- 1 tablespoon olive oil
- 2 sundried tomatoes, finely chopped
- 1 tablespoon prepared pesto sauce
- Sea salt and freshly ground pepper, to taste

Bring stock to a boil and add the couscous. Cover and remove from heat. Set aside for about 5 minutes.

Coat the shrimp with the egg and dredge in the breadcrumbs.

In a large sauté pan, heat the olive oil and add the shrimp, cooking until just brown and crispy on all sides.

Remove the lid to the couscous, then stir in the sundried tomatoes and pesto.

Season with sea salt and freshly ground pepper.

To stuff the shrimp, slice the front of the shrimp open and spoon the couscous mixture inside.

Serve with leftover couscous on the side.

Serves 2.

Mini Lettuce Wraps

Like a Greek salad wrapped in lettuce, this bite-sized appetizer is easy to assemble. Swap out the tomatoes, cucumbers, and red onion for any vegetables you like. Serve the wraps on their own or as part of a larger selection of appetizers.

- 1 tomato, diced
- 1 cucumber, diced
- 1 red onion, sliced
- 1 ounce low-fat feta cheese, crumbled
- Juice of 1 lemon
- 1 tablespoon olive oil
- Sea salt and freshly ground pepper, to taste
- 12 small intact iceberg lettuce leaves

Combine the tomato, cucumber, onion, and feta in a bowl with the lemon juice and olive oil.

Season with sea salt and freshly ground pepper.

Without tearing the leaves, gently fill each leaf with a tablespoon of the veggie mixture.

Roll them as tightly as you can, and lay them seam-side-down on a serving platter.

Makes about 1 dozen wraps.

Grilled Chicken Salad Pita

Tender and juicy grilled chicken topped with fresh vegetables in a pita pocket makes a filling and hearty meal. Serve this with celery and carrot sticks on the side for crunch instead of salty chips.

- 1 boneless, skinless chicken breast
- Sea salt and freshly ground pepper, to taste
- 1 cup baby spinach
- 1 roasted red pepper, sliced
- 1 tomato, chopped
- 1/2 small red onion, thinly sliced
- 1/2 small cucumber, chopped
- 4 tablespoons olive oil
- Juice of 1 lemon
- 1 whole-wheat pita pocket
- 2 tablespoons crumbled feta cheese

Preheat a gas or charcoal grill to medium-high heat.

Season the chicken breast with sea salt and freshly ground pepper, and grill until cooked through, about 7–8 minutes per side. Allow chicken to rest for 5 minutes before slicing into strips.

While the chicken is cooking, put all the chopped vegetables into a medium-mixing bowl and season with sea salt and freshly ground pepper.

Chop the chicken into cubes and add to salad. Add the olive oil and lemon juice and toss well.

Stuff the mixture onto a pita pocket and top with the feta cheese. Serve immediately.

Serves 1.

Open-Faced Eggplant Parmesan Sandwich

Eggplant Parmesan is often deep fried, laden with high-fat cheese, and served with mounds of pasta. In this version, the eggplant is broiled before being topped with marinara and low-fat Parmesan cheese, and served on a slice of toasted whole-grain bread. Eat with a knife and fork!

- 1 small eggplant, sliced into 1/4-inch rounds
- Pinch sea salt
- 2 tablespoons olive oil
- Sea salt and freshly ground pepper, to taste

- 2 slices whole-grain bread, thickly cut and toasted
- 1 cup marinara sauce (no added sugar)
- 1/4 cup freshly grated low-fat Parmesan cheese

Preheat broiler to high heat.

Salt both sides of the sliced eggplant, and let sit for 20 minutes to draw out the bitter juices.

Rinse the eggplant and pat dry with a paper towel. Brush the eggplant with the olive oil, and season with sea salt and freshly ground pepper.

Lay the eggplant on a sheet pan, and broil until crisp, about 4 minutes. Flip over and crisp the other side.

Lay the toasted bread on a sheet pan. Spoon some marinara sauce on each slice of bread, and layer the eggplant on top.

Sprinkle half of the cheese on top of the eggplant, top with more marinara sauce, and sprinkle with remaining cheese.

Put the sandwiches under the broiler until the cheese has melted, about 2 minutes. Using a spatula, transfer the sandwiches to plates and serve.

Serves 2.

Slow-Roasted Tomato and Basil Panini

Slow roasting tomatoes brings out their flavor, and cooking them actually increases their lycopene. Here the flavors of an Italian Caprese salad are transformed into a sandwich. If you don't have a panini maker or grill pan, you can easily toast the sandwich in a nonstick skillet.

- 4 Roma tomatoes, halved
- 4 cloves garlic
- 2 tablespoons olive oil
- 1 tablespoon Italian seasoning
- Sea salt and freshly ground pepper, to taste
- 4 basil leaves
- 2 slices fresh mozzarella
- 4 slices whole-grain bread

Preheat oven to 250 degrees.

Lay the tomatoes and garlic cloves on a sheet pan, and drizzle with the olive oil. Sprinkle with Italian seasoning, and season with the sea salt and freshly ground pepper.

Roast for about 2 1/2–3 hours, until tomatoes are extremely fragrant and slightly wilted.

To make the panini, layer the tomatoes with the basil and cheese on the bread. Preheat a panini maker, and cook the sandwiches until the bread is browned and the cheese is melted.

If you don't have a panini maker, just heat a grill pan on medium-high heat, and place your sandwich directly on the grill pan. Place another pan on top to press the sandwich.

Flip the panini after 3–4 minutes when the bread has nice grill marks, and cook the other side.

Serve warm.

Serves 2.

DINNER

Chances are that homemade dinner is either rare or rushed in your home. It's also typically the largest and heaviest meal on the American diet, but on the Mediterranean diet, try to make lunch the heavier meal whenever possible. Also be sure to have a cool glass of water and an apple or other fiber-rich snack about an hour before dinner to make having a light meal easier. This is especially important if you're eating with others not following the Mediterranean diet, and you will be forgoing their main entrée and sticking to a salad or a few sides.

Principles for the Evening Meal

Unless you're eating dinner early or planning on working out in the evening, you need far fewer carbs at your evening meal. Go easy on breads and pastas and load your plate with veggies and a small amount of protein.

Focus on filling your plate with about 50 percent plant foods, 25 percent grains, and 25 percent protein.

If possible, eat the Mediterranean way, with several small courses, such as a small salad, a cup of soup, an entrée, and a small dessert.

Make dinner a joyful, laughter-filled meal with friends and family, a quiet, intimate meal for two, or a lovely and special meal for one. The key is to make it special, no matter what night it is or how much company you have. Use candles, flowers, and your favorite dishes.

Linger at the table for as long as your family schedule will allow. Take your time with each course.

Meals for One

If you're dining alone, you have a lot more freedom and probably a lot more time to enjoy the preparation and the meal itself. Refrigerate extra dinner portions for lunch tomorrow, or freeze portions in small, microwaveable containers for another night.

If you can, avoid the temptation to read or watch TV during your meal. Really enjoy what's in front of you.

Meals with Family

Cooking Mediterranean-friendly meals when you're feeding non-dieting family members can be challenging. Most people are too busy or too tired in the evening to cook a separate meal for themselves. If you're not preparing something that works for both the family and your diet, have a snack an hour or so before dinner and stick to a salad and whatever veggies you're serving the family. If the family is having a meat or poultry entrée, set one portion aside before adding it to a casserole or dousing it in sauce, and chop it into a nice healthful salad.

There are plenty of meals that will work for both your diet and your family's palates. After trying these recipes, you'll have a repertoire that works for everyone.

Flank Steak and Blue Cheese Wraps

This snack or lunch dish uses leftover flank steak. Heat the flank steak if you like, or serve it cold. To boost the nutrition of these wraps, add fresh spinach leaves.

- 1 cup leftover flank steak, cut into 1-inch slices
- 1/4 cup red onion, thinly sliced
- 1/4 cup cherry tomatoes, chopped
- 1/4 cup low-salt olives, pitted and chopped
- 1/4 cup roasted red bell peppers, drained and coarsely chopped
- 1/4 cup blue cheese crumbles
- 6 whole-wheat or spinach wraps
- Sea salt and freshly ground pepper, to taste

Combine the flank steak, onion, tomatoes, olives, bell pepper, and blue cheese in a small bowl.

Spread 1/2 cup of this mixture on each wrap, and roll halfway. Fold the end in, and finish rolling like a burrito.

Cut on a diagonal if you'd like, season to taste, and serve.

Serves 6.

Spicy Broccoli Pasta Salad

Broccoli can help lower cholesterol, and it's high in vitamins C and K, as well as folate. This salad is perfect for picnics or potlucks.

- 8 ounces whole-wheat pasta
- 2 cups broccoli florets
- 1 cup carrots, peeled and shredded
- 1/4 cup plain Greek yogurt
- Juice of 1 lemon
- 1 teaspoon red pepper flakes
- Sea salt and freshly ground pepper, to taste

Cook the pasta according to the package directions for al dente and drain well.

When the pasta is cool, combine it with the veggies, yogurt, lemon juice, and red pepper flakes in a large bowl, and stir thoroughly to combine.

Taste for seasoning, and add sea salt and freshly ground pepper as needed.

Dish can be served at room temperature or chilled.

Serves 2.

Lamb and Vegetable Bake

This Greek-inspired one-dish meal combines lamb with a variety of garden vegetables. Improvise with the vegetables available in your garden or at your local farmers' market, but to maintain the authentic flavor, don't change the seasonings.

- 1/4 cup olive oil
- 1 pound boneless lean lamb, cut into 1/2-inch pieces
- 2 large red potatoes, scrubbed and diced
- 1 large onion, coarsely chopped
- 2 cloves garlic, minced
- 1 (28-ounce) can diced tomatoes with liquid (no salt added)
- 2 medium zucchini, cut into 1/2-inch slices
- 1 red bell pepper, seeded and cut into 1-inch cubes
- 2 tablespoons flat-leaf parsley, chopped
- 1 teaspoon dried thyme
- 1 tablespoon paprika
- 1/2 teaspoon ground cinnamon
- 1/2 cup red wine
- Sea salt and freshly ground pepper, to taste

Preheat the oven to 325 degrees.

Heat the olive oil in a large stew pot or cast-iron skillet over medium-high heat.

Add the lamb and brown the meat, stirring frequently. Transfer the lamb to an ovenproof baking dish.

Cook the potatoes, onion, and garlic in the skillet until tender, then transfer them to the baking dish.

Pour the tomatoes, zucchini, and pepper into the pan along with the herbs and spices, and simmer for 10 minutes.

Cover the lamb, onions, and potatoes with the tomato and pepper sauce and wine.

Cover with aluminum foil and bake for 1 hour. Uncover during the last 15 minutes of baking.

Season to taste, and serve with a green salad.

Serves 8.

Wild Mushroom Risotto

Risotto is a type of Italian starchy rice dish that cooks into a creamy consistency. It is classically paired with earthy wild mushrooms and Parmesan cheese. Serve it as a first course, or as a side dish with chicken or pork.

- 2 ounces dried porcini mushrooms
- 5 cups chicken stock
- 2 tablespoons olive oil
- 1 small onion, minced
- 2 cups brown rice
- 1/2 cup freshly grated low-fat Parmesan cheese
- Sea salt and freshly ground pepper, to taste

Place the mushrooms in a bowl and cover them with hot water. Set them aside for 30 minutes. Drain them, reserving the liquid, and wash them.

Strain the liquid through a sieve lined with cheesecloth. Add the liquid to the chicken stock.

Heat the chicken stock and mushroom liquid in a small saucepan. When simmering, turn heat to lowest setting.

Heat the olive oil in a large saucepan over medium heat. Add the onion and sauté for 3–5 minutes, or until tender. Stir in the rice and mushrooms and 3/4 cup of the stock.

Continue cooking the rice, stirring almost constantly, and adding more liquid, a ladleful at a time, as soon as the rice absorbs the liquid. There should always be some liquid visible in the pan. Cook, adding liquid every few minutes, until the rice is tender, with a slightly firm center, 20–30 minutes.

Remove from the heat, and stir in the Parmesan cheese, a spoonful at a time.

Season to taste and serve.

Serves 6.

Braised Duck with Fennel Root

Roasted or braised fennel is sweet and mild, and fennel provides a great source of vitamin C, fiber, and potassium. It pairs perfectly with the rich taste of duck, but you can also use chicken, which is leaner and lower in calories.

- 1/4 cup olive oil
- 1 whole duck, cleaned
- 3 teaspoon fresh rosemary
- 2 garlic cloves, minced
- Sea salt and freshly ground pepper, to taste
- 3 fennel bulbs, cut into chunks
- 1/2 cup sherry

Preheat the oven to 375 degrees.

Heat the olive oil in a large stew pot or Dutch oven.

Season the duck, including the cavity, with the rosemary, garlic, sea salt, and freshly ground pepper. Place the duck in the oil, and cook it for 10–15 minutes, turning as necessary to brown all sides.

Add the fennel bulbs and cook an additional 5 minutes.

Pour the sherry over the duck and fennel, cover the pot, and cook in the oven for 30–45 minutes, or until internal temperature of the duck is 140–150 degrees at its thickest part.

Allow duck to sit for 15 minutes before serving.

Serves 6.

Grilled Eggplant Pesto Stack

This pretty stack is inspired by the flavors of Italy. Making pesto is a cinch, although the store-bought variety will work if you're looking to make this dish fast. Eggplant is hearty enough to be a great meat substitute.

For the pesto:
- 1 large bunch basil, or 1 cup tightly packed basil leaves
- 1/2 cup pine nuts, toasted
- 2–3 cloves garlic
- Juice of 1 lime
- 3/4 cup olive oil
- 1/2 cup freshly grated low-fat Parmesan cheese
- Sea salt and freshly ground pepper, to taste

For the eggplant:
- 1 medium eggplant, sliced into 1/2-inch thick slices
- 2 tablespoons olive oil

Make the pesto:

Put the basil, pine nuts, garlic, and lime juice in a food processor, and pulse until you have a thick paste.

Continue to pulse and slowly drizzle in the olive oil until you have a creamy sauce.

Fold in the cheese unless you plan to freeze the pesto.

Season with sea salt and freshly ground pepper.

Make the eggplant:

Preheat a grill to medium-high heat.

Salt the eggplant and let rest for 20 minutes to get the bitter juices out. Rinse the eggplant and pat dry with a paper towel.

Brush the eggplant with 2 tablespoons olive oil, and lay on the grill. Grill for 5–6 minutes per side, until the eggplant is lightly charred but still firm.

To serve, layer the grilled eggplant with the pesto on individual plates.

Serves 4.

Chicken Tagine with Olives

Tagine is a traditional Moroccan stew. This version gets its bright color from saffron and turmeric. Use a combination of purple and green pitted olives if you can find them. Olives are a key component of the Mediterranean diet, and are a good source of vitamin E.

- 1 teaspoon ground ginger
- 1/2 teaspoon ground cumin
- 1/2 teaspoon paprika
- 1/2 teaspoon turmeric
- Pinch saffron threads
- 1 clove garlic, minced
- 1 whole chicken
- 2 medium onions, thinly sliced
- 1/2 cup finely chopped flat-leaf parsley
- 1/2 cup finely chopped cilantro

- 1 cinnamon stick
- 3 cups water
- 2 tablespoons olive oil
- 1 tablespoon butter
- Juice and zest of 1 lemon
- 1 cup green or purple olives (or a combination of both), pitted
- Sea salt and freshly ground pepper, to taste

Combine the spices and garlic in a small bowl.

Pat the chicken dry, brush the spices over the chicken, and massage it in with your fingers, including in the cavity.

Place the chicken in a large stew pot or Dutch oven. Add the onions, parsley, cilantro, and cinnamon stick to the pot along with the water. Bring the water to a boil and add the olive oil, butter, and lemon zest and juice.

Cover and simmer for 1–2 hours, or until the chicken is tender and the sauce has reduced and thickened slightly.

Remove the lid and simmer an additional 15 minutes. Season with sea salt and freshly ground pepper to taste.

Add the olives immediately before serving.

Serves 6.

Quinoa, Broccoli, and Baby Potatoes

Originally from the Andes, quinoa is a starch that's quick and easy to cook as well as extremely healthful: it's high in manganese, magnesium, protein, and more. Before cooking quinoa be sure to rinse it; otherwise, it may have a bitter flavor.

- 2 tablespoons olive oil
- 1 cup baby potatoes, cut in half
- 1 cup broccoli florets
- 2 cups cooked quinoa
- Zest of 1 lemon
- Sea salt and freshly ground pepper, to taste

Heat the olive oil in a large skillet.

Add the potatoes and cook until tender and golden brown.

Add the broccoli and cook until soft, about 3 minutes.

Remove from heat and add the quinoa and lemon zest. Season and serve.

Serves 4.

Shrimp Salad

Main dish salads are a great way to get many servings of vegetables in one meal. Serve this tasty fare with whole-wheat pita bread for a light lunch or dinner.

For the vinaigrette:
- 1/8 cup red wine vinegar
- Juice of 1 lemon
- 1 small shallot, finely minced
- 1 tablespoon fresh mint, chopped
- 1/4 teaspoon dried oregano
- 1/4 cup olive oil
- Sea salt and freshly ground pepper, to taste

For the salad:
- 1 pound shrimp, deveined and shelled
- Juice and zest of 1 lemon
- 1 clove garlic, minced
- 2 cups baby spinach leaves
- 1 cup romaine lettuce, chopped
- 1/2 cup grape tomatoes
- 1 medium cucumber, peeled, seeded, and diced
- 1/2 cup low-salt olives, pitted
- 1/4 cup low-fat feta cheese

Make the vinaigrette:

Combine the wine vinegar, lemon juice, shallot, chopped mint, and oregano in a bowl.

Add the olive oil, whisking constantly for up to 1 minute, or until you create a smooth emulsion, then season with sea salt and freshly ground pepper.

Refrigerate for 1 hour and whisk before serving if separated.

Make the salad:

Combine the shrimp with the lemon juice and garlic in a shallow bowl or bag. Marinate for at least 2 hours.

Grill the shrimp in a grill basket or sauté in a frying pan for 2–3 minutes until pink.

In a large bowl, toss the greens, tomatoes, cucumber, olives, and feta cheese together. Toss the shrimp with the salad mixture, and drizzle with the vinaigrette.

Serve immediately.

Serves 4.

Roast Pork Tenderloin

By simply altering the seasonings slightly, this traditional pork tenderloin takes on a decidedly Spanish flair. Remember, the diet allows red meat once per week. Serve it with red potatoes, or add it to salads, wraps, or sandwiches.

- 2 tablespoons olive oil
- 1 teaspoon Spanish paprika
- 1 teaspoon red wine vinegar
- 1 clove garlic, minced
- 1/2 teaspoon ground cumin
- 1/2 teaspoon ground coriander
- 1/2 teaspoon ginger
- 1/2 teaspoon freshly ground pepper
- 1/4 teaspoon turmeric
- 1 pound pork tenderloin
- Sea salt and freshly ground pepper, to taste

Combine all the ingredients except the pork tenderloin.

Spread over the meat in a thick paste, cover, and refrigerate for several hours or overnight.

Heat a grill to medium heat, and grill the tenderloin for 10–12 minutes, turning halfway through. An instant-read thermometer should read 145 degrees.

Transfer the meat to a serving platter, and allow it to rest for 15 minutes before slicing.

Season to taste and serve.

Serves 6.

Roasted Balsamic Brussels Sprouts with Pecans

This is a terrific recipe for those who say they don't like Brussels sprouts, as roasting them brings out their sweetness. The vinegar helps by adding a tart flavor as well, and will make getting your daily requirement of vegetables a breeze. Substitute walnuts or almonds for the pecans, if you prefer.

- 20–25 medium-sized Brussels sprouts, quartered
- 2 tablespoons olive oil
- 1 tablespoon balsamic vinegar
- Sea salt and freshly ground pepper, to taste
- 1/4 cup chopped pecans, toasted

Preheat oven to 400 degrees.

Spread sprouts on a single layer on a baking sheet.

Drizzle with olive oil, vinegar, sea salt, and freshly ground pepper.

Roast for 15–20 minutes until tender and caramelized.

Top with the toasted pecans and serve.

Serves 4.

Baked Salmon with Capers and Olives

This fresh-tasting salmon dish is inspired by the cuisine of Greece and Italy. Salmon is a great source of omega-3 fatty acids.

- 1 tablespoon olive oil, divided
- 4 salmon steaks
- Sea salt and freshly ground pepper, to taste
- 2 Roma tomatoes, chopped
- 1/4 cup green olives, pitted and chopped
- 1 clove garlic, minced
- Juice of 1/2 lemon
- 1 teaspoon capers, rinsed and drained
- 1/2 teaspoon sugar
- 1/2 cup dry breadcrumbs

Preheat the oven to 375 degrees.

Brush a baking dish with the olive oil. Place the salmon steaks in the dish.

Season with sea salt and freshly ground pepper.

In a large bowl, combine all the remaining ingredients.

Top the salmon steaks with the tomato mixture, then the breadcrumbs.

Drizzle with the remaining olive oil and bake for 15 minutes, or until medium rare.

Serves 4.

Rosemary-Roasted Acorn Squash

When roasted at high heat, the skin of acorn squash becomes soft, tender, and edible. Meanwhile, the benefits of rosemary are many: it is thought to stimulate the immune system, increase circulation, and improve digestion.

- 1 acorn squash
- 2 tablespoons honey
- 2 tablespoons rosemary, finely chopped
- 2 tablespoons olive oil
- Sea salt, to taste

Preheat oven to 400 degrees.

Cut squash in half, and clean out the seeds.

Slice each half into 4 wedges.

Mix honey, rosemary, and olive oil.

Lay squash on baking sheet, and sprinkle each slice with a bit of the mixture and a touch of sea salt. Turn over and sprinkle other side.

Bake for 30 minutes or so until squash is tender and slightly caramelized, turning each slice over halfway through.

Serve immediately.

Serves 4.

Clam Spaghetti

Nothing could be simpler for a weeknight meal than this easy pasta dish. Clams are rich in iron, protein, omega-3 fatty acids, and vitamin B12. Leave out the bacon if you are trying to cut calories.

- 1/4 cup olive oil
- 4 ounces bacon
- 1 medium onion, diced
- 1 medium green pepper, seeded and diced
- 4 garlic cloves, minced
- 1/2 cup flat-leaf parsley, chopped
- 1/3 teaspoon cayenne pepper
- Sea salt and freshly ground pepper, to taste
- 3 dozen or so clams, depending on their size
- 1/2 cup white wine
- 1 pound whole-wheat spaghetti
- 1 lemon, cut into wedges
- 1/2 cup freshly grated low-fat Parmesan cheese

Heat the olive oil in a large skillet over medium heat.

Add the bacon, onion, pepper, and garlic, and cook until the bacon is slightly crisp and the onion is translucent.

Add the parsley, cayenne pepper, sea salt, and freshly ground pepper, and set aside.

Bring a pot of water to a boil. Add the clams and boil for 10 minutes, or until they open. Remove the clams from the pot, and shell half of them.

Return the skillet to medium-high heat.

Add the shelled clams to the skillet, along with the remaining clams, white wine, and 2 cups of the liquid used to boil the clams.

Cook the pasta according to package directions for al dente, and place in a large serving dish.

Ladle the clam and bacon mixture over the pasta, and toss to serve.

Garnish with lemon wedges and Parmesan cheese.

Serves 4.

Halibut with Roasted Vegetables

Halibut is a firm, mild fish that pairs well with a variety of seasonings and vegetables. Here, it's combined with tomatoes and zucchini—traditional Mediterranean vegetables—but feel free to improvise with what's available in your garden or farmers' market.

- 1/4 cup small white mushrooms, coarsely chopped
- 2 small tomatoes, coarsely chopped
- 1 small white onion, chopped
- 2 zucchini, chopped
- 2 cloves garlic, minced
- 1 teaspoon Herbes de Provence
- 1/2 cup olive oil
- Sea salt and freshly ground pepper, to taste
- 1 1/2 pounds halibut steak, cut into 6 pieces
- 3 tablespoons fresh tarragon, chopped finely
- Juice of 1 lemon

Preheat the oven to 350 degrees.

Toss the vegetables and herbs on a large baking sheet with the olive oil, and season with sea salt and freshly ground pepper. Roast for 15–20 minutes, or until soft and slightly browned.

Place the halibut steaks on another baking sheet, and season with the tarragon, sea salt, freshly ground pepper, and lemon juice. Roast for 10–13 minutes.

Top the halibut steaks with the roasted vegetables.

Serves 6.

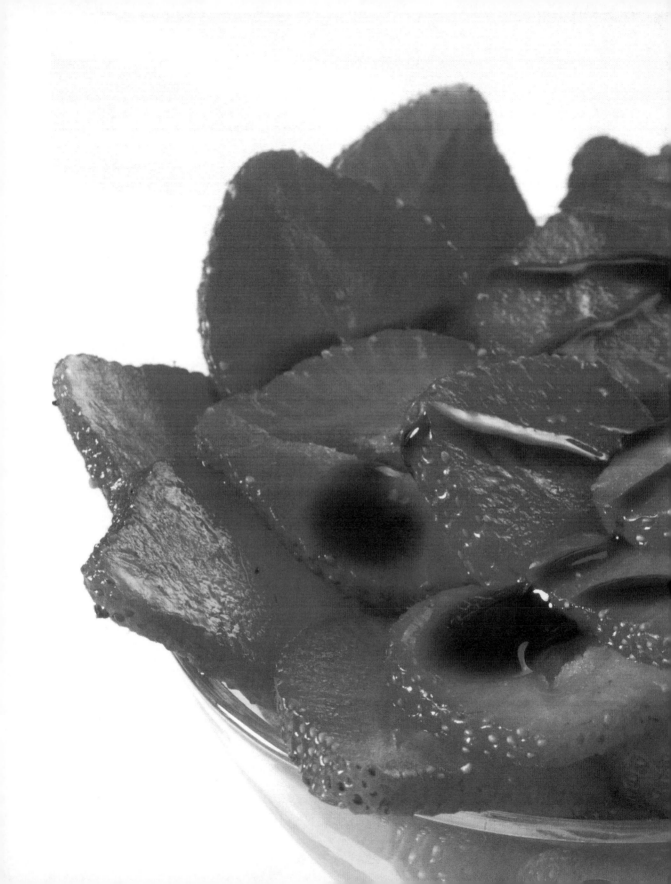

DESSERT

Americans like their desserts and sweets. Many can't imagine a meal without some type of dessert. Dessert as Americans know it is a relatively rare thing to Europeans and Mediterranean peoples. In these regions, dessert is often a small plate of cheeses, nuts, or fruit. This is a delicious and terrifically healthful way to end a meal, but if you're having trouble adjusting your idea of dessert, try not to beat yourself up. As your palate and your stomach become accustomed to a healthier diet, your cravings for cookies, cakes, full-fat ice cream, and other diet saboteurs will diminish.

Don't Deprive Yourself, Reward Yourself!

Until then, remember that the Mediterranean diet isn't meant to make you feel deprived or unfulfilled; you're supposed to feel joyous and satisfied. If you absolutely can't live without your friends Ben and Jerry, don't. Just limit their visits to once or twice a month and buy the smallest container at the store, so that leftovers won't be the end of you.

It's okay to reward yourself with a sweet cheat once in a while to celebrate a month of healthful eating or a weight loss goal that's been reached. Better yet, choose non-food rewards, such as new clothing or a favorite author's new book. The important thing with food-related rewards is to plan, limit, and savor them. If you binge or give in to unplanned cravings, you'll get discouraged and likely lose some motivation.

Greek Yogurt and Marinated Pineapple

This recipe is a quick and easy dessert that's just as nutritious as it is tasty. The Greek yogurt has a healthful serving of protein, and the enzymes in pineapple aid digestion. The pineapple can be prepared up to three days ahead and is actually better when it's allowed to marinate overnight.

• 1 cup fresh pineapple, diced	• 1 tablespoon fresh crushed mint
• 1/4 cup unsweetened pineapple juice	• 1 teaspoon honey
• 1 tablespoon fresh lemon juice	• 2 cups vanilla Greek yogurt
• 1 teaspoon lemon zest	• Additional fresh mint leaves for garnish

In a small bowl, combine the pineapple, pineapple juice, lemon juice, lemon zest, crushed mint, and honey. Mix well.

Spoon into a quart-sized zippered plastic bag and shake a few times after sealing. Allow to marinate in the fridge for at least 4 hours, preferably overnight, shaking gently 2–3 times during marinating time.

Spoon 1/2 cup of Greek yogurt into dessert dishes and top with 1/4 cup of the pineapple topping. Garnish with fresh mint leaves, if desired.

Serves 4.

Orange and Whipped-Cheese Dessert Cups

Although this dessert is very simple to make, it tastes decadent and is pretty to look at. This makes it a great dessert to serve to guests or after a romantic dinner for two. The taste is similar to cheesecake, but with a creamier texture and a good deal less sugar.

- 1 cup part-skim ricotta cheese
- 1 cup low-fat cream cheese
- 2 tablespoons honey
- 2 tablespoons low-fat milk
- 1/2 teaspoon vanilla
- 1/2 teaspoon cinnamon
- 2 teaspoons honey
- 1/2 teaspoon allspice
- 1/4 teaspoon nutmeg
- 3 large navel oranges, sectioned, membrane removed
- Fresh basil leaves for garnish

In a blender or food processor, combine the ricotta, cream cheese, honey, milk, vanilla, and cinnamon, and process until smooth.

Spoon into four dessert cups, cover, and refrigerate.

In a medium-sized heavy skillet, heat the honey until thin and warm. Stir in the allspice and nutmeg until well mixed.

Add the orange slices and cook for 1 minute. Gently turn the orange slices over and cook for 1–2 minutes or until just beginning to brown. Remove from heat.

Allow the orange slices to cool to room temperature, then top each dessert dish with 1/4 of the oranges. To serve, garnish with a basil leaf.

Serves 4.

Fruit Kabobs with Dark Chocolate Drizzle

This dessert is very popular with kids and is a great one to serve at casual parties. If you prefer to serve the chocolate sauce fondue style, simply use a snack-sized slow cooker to keep the sauce warm and allow your guests to dip.

- 1 cantaloupe, peeled and cut into chunks
- 1 honeydew melon, peeled and cut into chunks
- 1 pound fresh strawberries, capped
- 8 bamboo skewers soaked 30 minutes in water

- 1 cup dark chocolate chips
- 1/2 cup milk
- 1 teaspoon vanilla

Preheat the broiler and line a baking sheet with aluminum foil.

Thread the fruit onto the skewers in an alternating pattern and place onto the baking sheet. Broil for 3 minutes, turn, and broil for an additional 2 minutes.

Meanwhile, heat the milk in the microwave for about 90 seconds. Heat just until steaming but not foamy and boiled.

Place the chocolate chips into a large glass bowl and pour the milk over the chips. Add the vanilla and stir until smooth.

Remove the fruit kabobs from the oven and place on a platter. Drizzle with the chocolate sauce and serve.

Serves 4.

Red-Wine Poached Pears

Red wine is encouraged on this diet and is popular with meals in Italy, France, and Spain. Pears are a low-calorie fruit and a good source of fiber. These make a delicious dessert but are also lovely alongside rich meat dishes as well.

- 2 cups red wine, such as Merlot or Zinfandel, more if necessary
- 2 firm pears, peeled
- 2–3 cardamom pods, split
- 1 cinnamon stick
- 2 peppercorns
- 1 bay leaf

Put all ingredients in a large pot and bring to a boil.

Make sure the pears are submerged in the wine.

Reduce heat and simmer for 15–20 minutes until the pears are tender when poked with a fork. Remove the pears from the wine, and allow to cool.

Bring the wine to a boil, and cook until it reduces to a syrup.

Strain and drizzle the pears with the warmed syrup before serving.

Serves 2.

Balsamic Strawberries

Strawberries with balsamic vinegar is a classic Italian treat. This easy and unique way to eat fresh summer berries even works if the berries are not as flavorful as you might like. Allow the berries to macerate for a few minutes before serving.

- 2 cups strawberries, hulled and sliced
- 2 tablespoons sugar
- 2 tablespoons balsamic vinegar

Put the strawberries in a bowl, sprinkle with the sugar, and lightly drizzle with the balsamic vinegar.

Toss to combine and let sit for about 10 minutes before serving.

Serves 2.

Pears with Blue Cheese and Walnuts

Fruit, cheese, and nuts are a classic combination, regarding flavor but also health—walnuts provide a good source of omega-3 fatty acids, and pears are a good source of fiber. Enjoy this treat as a dessert or healthful snack.

- 1–2 pears, cored and sliced into 12 slices
- 1/4 cup blue cheese crumbles
- 12 walnut halves
- 1 tablespoon honey

Lay the pear slices on a plate, and top with the blue cheese crumbles.

Top each slice with 1 walnut, and drizzle with honey.

Serve and enjoy!

Serves 1.

Banana Cream Pie Parfaits

Low-fat vanilla pudding and graham cracker crumbs make this a simple and healthful treat, with walnuts and bananas providing potassium and omega-3 fatty acids. These parfaits can be prepared ahead of time, making this an easy dessert option for a picnic.

- 1 cup nonfat vanilla pudding
- 2 low-sugar graham crackers, crushed
- 1 banana, peeled and sliced
- 1/4 cup walnuts, chopped
- Honey for drizzling

In small parfait dishes or glasses, layer the ingredients, starting with the pudding and ending with chopped walnuts.

You can repeat the layers, depending on the size of the glass and your preferences.

Drizzle with the honey.

Serve chilled.

Serves 2.

Honey-Vanilla Apple Pie with Olive Oil Crust

Olive oil is the preferred cooking oil on the Mediterranean diet and can be used successfully in baking. The whole-wheat flour will give the pie a rustic appearance.

For the crust:

- 1/4 cup olive oil
- 1 1/2 cups whole-wheat flour
- 1/2 teaspoon sea salt
- 2 tablespoons ice water

For the filling:

- 4 large apples of your choice, peeled, cored, and sliced
- Juice of 1 lemon
- 1 tablespoon pure vanilla extract
- 1 tablespoon honey
- 1/2 teaspoon sea salt
- Olive oil

Make the crust:

Put the olive oil, flour, and sea salt in a food processor and process until dough forms.

Slowly add the water and pulse until you have a stiff dough.

Form the dough into 2 equal-sized balls, wrap in plastic wrap, and put in the refrigerator while you make the filling.

Make the filling:

Combine the apples, lemon juice, vanilla, honey, and sea salt in a large bowl.

Stir to combine and allow to sit for at least 10 minutes.

Preheat oven to 400 degrees.

Roll 1 crust out on a lightly floured surface. Transfer to a 9-inch pie plate and top with filling.

Roll the other ball of dough out and put on top of the pie. Cut a few slices in the top to vent the pie.

Lightly brush the top of the pie with olive oil.

Bake for 45 minutes, or until top is browned and apples are bubbly.

Allow to cool completely before slicing and serving with your favorite frozen yogurt.

Serves 8.

Berry Crumble

While this may seem like a decadent dessert, it's actually loaded with antioxidant-filled berries and cholesterol-lowering oats. If you don't have a cast-iron skillet, simply use a casserole dish instead. Use naturally sweet, ripe berries in this easy-to-make dessert.

- 3 cups frozen, mixed berries
- 1 cup rolled oats
- 2 tablespoons brown sugar
- 1 tablespoon whole-wheat flour
- 2 tablespoons margarine

Preheat oven to 400 degrees.

In a 10-inch, cast-iron skillet, lay the berries in an even layer.

Mix the oats with the sugar and flour in a large mixing bowl.

Spread the oat mixture evenly on top of the berries.

Crumble with the butter, and bake for 40–50 minutes until top is brown and berries are bubbly.

Serve warm.

Serves 6.

Grilled Stone Fruit

Juicy summer fruit provides hydration in addition to vitamins. These stone fruits are also delicious drizzled with balsamic vinegar instead of cheese and honey for a savory side dish.

- 2 peaches, halved and pitted
- 2 plums, halved and pitted
- 3 apricots, halved and pitted
- 1/2 cup low-fat ricotta cheese
- 2 tablespoons honey

Heat grill to medium heat.

Oil the grates or spray with cooking spray.

Place the fruit cut-side-down on the grill, and grill for 2–3 minutes per side, until lightly charred and soft.

Serve warm with the ricotta and drizzle with honey.

Serves 2.

Home-Baked Biscotti

Biscotti are a favorite sweet in Italy, particularly served alongside espresso. Happily, they're one of the easiest treats to bake. These keep well in an airtight container for up to two weeks, so double the recipe to make enough to last a while. These are also wonderful dipped in red wine.

- 2 cups whole-wheat flour
- 3/4 cup sugar
- 1 teaspoon baking powder
- 1/4 teaspoon salt
- 3/4 cup slivered almonds
- 3 large eggs
- 2 tablespoons pure almond extract
- 1 teaspoon pure vanilla extract
- 1 teaspoon extra-virgin olive oil

Place an oven rack in the middle position and preheat the oven to 275 degrees.

In a large bowl, combine the flour, sugar, baking powder, salt, and almonds and stir with a wooden spoon until well combined.

In a small bowl, whisk together the eggs, almond extract, and vanilla.

Pour the egg mixture into the dry ingredients and use a wooden spoon to mix well, stirring for about 2 minutes to ensure that the ingredients are well combined.

Use your hands to grease a baking sheet with the olive oil and then use your greased hands to spread the dough onto the baking sheet in a rectangle about 11 x 4 inches.

Bake for 45 minutes, remove from the oven, and use a sharp, greased knife to cut the rectangle crosswise into 1/2-inch slices. Separate the slices so that none are touching and return the baking sheet to the oven.

Bake until the cut sides are quite dry, about 20 minutes more.

Cool on the baking sheet to room temperature, then store in an airtight container.

Makes about 20 biscotti.

Frozen Raspberry Delight

You can make a sorbet-style treat with frozen fruit. While truly tasty, this dessert will also help you meet your daily fruit requirement. Swap the peach or mango for a banana, if you prefer.

- 3 cups frozen raspberries
- 1 peach, peeled and pitted
- 1 mango, peeled and pitted
- 1 teaspoon honey

Add all ingredients to a blender and puree, only adding enough water to keep the mixture moving and your blender from overworking itself.

Freeze for 10 minutes to firm up if desired.

Serves 2.

Cocoa and Coconut Banana Slices

Frozen bananas have a creamy consistency that mimics ice cream. Bananas are good for you, too—providing dietary fiber, vitamin C, potassium, and manganese. This dessert makes a great snack for adults and kids alike.

- 1 banana, peeled and sliced
- 2 tablespoons unsweetened shredded coconut
- 1 tablespoon unsweetened cocoa powder
- 1 teaspoon honey

Lay the banana slices on a parchment-lined baking sheet in a single layer.

Put in the freezer for about 10 minutes, until firm but not frozen solid.

Mix the coconut with the cocoa powder in a small bowl.

Roll the banana slices in honey, followed by the coconut mixture.

You can either eat immediately or put back in the freezer for a frozen, sweet treat.

Serves 1.

Fresh Figs with Chocolate Sauce

Desserts in the Mediterranean are simple and often fruity. This easy treat would be a good snack, too. You could also serve it with Greek yogurt.

- 1/4 cup honey
- 2 tablespoons cocoa powder

- 8 fresh figs

Combine the honey and cocoa powder in a small bowl, and mix well to form a syrup.

Cut the figs in half and place cut side up.

Drizzle with the syrup and serve.

Serves 4.

Cranberry-Orange Cheesecake Pears

For this fruity, creamy treat, use the lightest cream cheese you can find, or substitute low- or nonfat ricotta. On the other hand, pears are very nutritious, a good source of fiber, and low in calories. Finally the cranberries and almonds add flavor but can be swapped out for other dried fruit and nuts, if you prefer.

- 5 firm pears
- 1 cup unsweetened cranberry juice
- 1 cup freshly squeezed orange juice
- 1 tablespoon pure vanilla extract
- 1/2 teaspoon ground cinnamon
- 1/2 cup low-fat cream cheese, softened
- 1/4 teaspoon ground ginger
- 1/4 teaspoon almond extract
- 1/4 cup dried, unsweetened cranberries
- 1/4 cup sliced almonds, toasted

Peel the pears and slice off the bottoms so they sit upright. Remove the cores, and put the pears in a wide saucepan.

Add the cranberry and orange juice, as well as the vanilla and cinnamon extract. Bring to a boil, and reduce to a simmer. Cover and simmer on low heat for 25–30 minutes, until pears are soft but not falling apart.

Beat the cream cheese with the ginger and almond extract.

Stir the cranberries and almonds into the cream cheese mixture.

Once the pears have cooled, spoon the cream cheese into them.

Boil the remaining juices down to a syrup, and drizzle over the top of the filled pears.

Serves 5.

CONCLUSION

One of the hardest things about dieting and making healthful lifestyle changes is realizing that it isn't selfish, self-centered, or vain. This is especially difficult for parents, who spend a great deal of time nurturing and caring for their children and very little nurturing and caring for themselves.

However, without a healthy body and a healthy heart, you may not be able to care for, enjoy, and spend time with your loved ones the way you would like. You owe it to the people you love to take care of yourself the way you take care of them.

Just as importantly, you deserve to feel your best, to have the energy to pursue your interests and dreams, and to have the fitness to try new things and live each day to its fullest. You also deserve to feel confidant and attractive in your own skin.

A healthful diet such as the Mediterranean diet isn't just a tool to lose weight. It's a way to get everything out of life that it has to offer.

8652012R00065

Printed in Great Britain
by Amazon.co.uk, Ltd.,
Marston Gate.